Study Guide

Introduction to Clinical Pharmacology

Eighth Edition

Marilyn Winterton Edmunds, PhD, ANP/GNP

Adjunct Faculty
Johns Hopkins University
School of Nursing
Baltimore, Maryland

ELSEVIER
MOSBY

ELSEVIER
MOSBY

3251 Riverport Lane
St. Louis, Missouri 63043

STUDY GUIDE FOR INTRODUCTION TO
CLINICAL PHARMACOLOGY, Eighth Edition   ISBN: 978-0-323-18900-2

Senior Content Strategist: Nancy O'Brien
Developmental Editor: Heather Rippetoe
Publishing Services Manager: Jeff Patterson
Design Direction: Karen Pauls

Printed in the United States of America

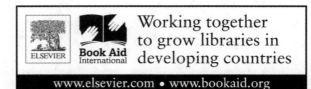

Working together
to grow libraries in
developing countries

www.elsevier.com • www.bookaid.org

Last digit is the print number: 9 8 7 6 5 4 3 2

Reviewers

Jacqueline Rosenjack Burchum, DNSc, FNP-BC, CNE
Associate Professor
Health Science Center
University of Tennessee
Memphis, Tennessee

Drew Case, MSN
Instructor
Doane College
School of Graduate and Professional Studies
Lincoln, Nebraska

T. Camille Lindsey Killough RN, BSN
Instructor
Nursing Department
Pearl River Community College
Hattiesburg, Mississippi

Sallie Noto RN, MS, MSN
Retired
Career Technology Center
School of Practical Nursing
Scranton, Pennsylvania

To the Student

The role of the LPN/LVN is becoming increasingly important in the health care system, particularly as many registered nurses retire and leave the profession. More and more LPN/LVNs will move into responsible positions in a wide variety of settings—both inside and outside the US—where this book is used. LPN/LVNs must be prepared to practice in settings with advanced technology, many other health care workers, and increasingly complex patients, diseases, and treatments. They must also be prepared to care for patients in areas where they may be one of the only health care workers; where there is no technology; and many challenging patients, diseases, and treatments.

This textbook was written in a concise and simple manner to share important information about the complex process of administering medications. It was written deliberately to provide information that LPN/LVNs must know. The Study Guide is designed to help those students who are serious about doing well on the NCLEX exams and caring well for patients. The content has been selected based on what faculty from a variety of LPN/LVN programs agree is relevant and necessary.

Learning about pharmacology and the medications to give to your patients is important. Mastering difficult concepts and tasks is often a great source of personal happiness.

Marilyn Winterton Edmunds, PhD, ANP/GNP
Adjunct Faculty
Johns Hopkins University
School of Nursing
Baltimore, Maryland

STUDY HINTS FOR ALL STUDENTS

Ask Questions!

There are no stupid questions. If you do not know something or are not sure, you need to find out. Other people may be wondering the same thing, but may be too shy to ask. The answer could mean life or death to your patient. That is certainly more important than feeling embarrassed about asking a question.

Chapter Objectives

At the beginning of each chapter in the textbook are objectives that you should have mastered when you finish studying that chapter. Write these objectives in your notebook, leaving a blank space after each. Fill in the answers as you find them while reading the chapter. Review to make sure your answers are correct and complete. Use these answers when you study for tests. This should also be done for separate course objectives that your instructor has listed in your class syllabus.

Evolve Website

The evolve website to accompany the *Introduction to Clinical Pharmacology*, 8th edition textbook contains the following resources: Animations; Answer Keys to case studies, critical thinking questions and end of chapter NCLEX Review Questions; Drug Dosage Calculators; an audio and English/Spanish glossary; Interactive NCLEX Review Questions; Patient Teaching Handouts; Videoclips; and weblinks. Using these resources as you study can help you master the material. The Evolve website for the textbook can be found at (http://evolve.elsevier.com/Edmunds/LPN/).

Key Terms

At the beginning of each chapter in the textbook are key terms that you will encounter as you read the chapter. Text page number references are provided for easy reference and review, and the key terms are in color the first time they appear in the chapter. Phonetic pronunciations are provided for terms that you might find difficult to pronounce. The goal is to help the student reader with limited proficiency in English to develop a greater command of the pronunciation of scientific and nonscientific terminology in English. It is hoped that a more general competency in the understanding and use of medical and scientific language may result.

Key Points

Use the Key Points at the end of each chapter in the textbook to help with review for exams.

Reading Hints

When reading each chapter in the textbook, look at the subject headings to learn what each section is about. Read for the general meaning first. Then reread parts you did not understand. It may help to read those parts aloud. Carefully read the information given in each table and study each figure and its caption.

Concepts

While studying, put difficult concepts into your own words to see if you understand them. Check this understanding with another student or the instructor. Write these in your notebook.

Class Notes

When taking lecture notes in class, leave a large margin on the left side of each notebook page and write only on right-hand pages, leaving all left-hand pages blank. Look over your lecture notes soon after each class, while your memory is fresh. Fill in missing words, complete sentences and ideas, and underline key phrases, definitions, and concepts. At the top of each page, write the topic of that page. In the left margin, write the key word for that part of your notes. On the opposite left-hand page, write a summary or outline that combines material from both the textbook and the lecture. These can be your study notes for review.

Study Groups

Form a study group with other students so you can help each other. Practice speaking and reading aloud. Ask questions about material you are not sure about. Work together to find answers. Attempt to answer the textbook and syllabus objectives in your own words.

References for Improving Study Skills

Good study skills are essential for achieving your goals in nursing. Time management, efficient use of study time, and a consistent approach to studying are all beneficial. There are various study methods for reading a textbook and for taking class notes. Some methods that have proven helpful can be found in *Saunders Student Nurse Planner* by Susan deWit. This book contains helpful information on test-taking and preparing for clinical experiences. It includes an example of a "time map" for planning study time and a blank form that you can use to formulate a personal time map.

ADDITIONAL STUDY HINTS FOR ESL/LEP (ENGLISH AS A SECOND-LANGUAGE/LIMITED ENGLISH PROFICIENCY) STUDENTS

First Language Buddy

ESL/LEP students should find a first-language buddy—another student who is a native speaker of English and is willing to answer questions about word meanings, pronunciations, and culture. Maybe your buddy would like to learn about your language and culture too. This could help in his or her nursing experience as well.

Vocabulary

If you find a nontechnical word you do not know (e.g., *drowsy*), try to guess its meaning from the sentence (e.g., *With electrolyte imbalance, the patient may feel fatigued and drowsy.*). If you are not sure of the meaning, or if it seems particularly important, look it up in the dictionary. (If you guessed that *drowsy* means something like sleepy, you were correct!). If there is a technical word you do not understand or remember, look for it in the index at the back of the textbook or in your medical dictionary. Write it in your notebook. Keep an alphabetical list of words you have difficulty remembering so you can look them up easily and review them before a test.

Vocabulary Notebook

Keep a small alphabetized notebook or address book in your pocket or purse. Write down new nontechnical words you read or hear along with their meanings and pronunciations. Write each word under its initial letter so you can find it easily, as in a dictionary. For words you do not know or for words that have a different meaning in nursing, write down how they sound and are used. Look up their meanings in a dictionary or ask your instructor or first-language buddy. Then write the different meanings or usages that you have found in your book, including the nursing meaning. Continue to add new words as you discover them. For example:

primary
- of most importance; main: *the primary problem or disease*
- **the first one; elementary:** *primary school*

secondary
- of less importance; resulting from another problem or disease: *a secondary symptom*
- **the second one:** *secondary school* (in the United States, high school)

Student Name_____ Date_____

Pharmacology and the Nursing Process in LPN Practice

chapter

1

 Go to http://evolve.elsevier.com/edmunds/lpn/ for additional activities and exercises.

PART I: SUBJECTIVE AND OBJECTIVE INFORMATION

1. The steps in the nursing process involve talking to the patient and collecting information about the medications he or she takes. Place the following steps of the nursing process in the order in which they are generally performed.
   1. implementation
   2. diagnosis
   3. assessment
   4. evaluation
   5. planning
   _____, _____, _____, _____, _____

2. Give examples of some of the things the LPN/LVN might do in each of the five steps of the nursing process. Do you feel that some of these steps are more important than others? Would the importance of the steps differ because of the type of drug being given (for example, a drug for a heart problem vs. an antibiotic)? Think about these things and discuss your answers with your classmates.

3. The six rights of medication administration are important to know. Identify the six rights from the list. *(Select all that apply.)*
   1. right patient
   2. right abbreviations
   3. right dose
   4. right medication
   5. right formula
   6. right documentation
   7. right route
   8. right time
   9. right doctor

4. LPN/LVNs have learned to use the nursing process in providing basic care. It is also used in giving the patient medications. To give medications safely, the nurse has to pay attention to both the process and the patient. From the case study below, underline some of the things that you believe are important for the LPN/LVN to note.

   A 56-year-old man came into the ambulatory clinic complaining of chest pain. He states that after eating lunch he noticed an excess of gas and pain in his chest that he thought was heartburn. After a few minutes the pain got worse, and he felt dizzy. His heart felt like it was racing, and he started to perspire and to feel nauseated. The nurse took his vital signs: heart rate 120, blood pressure 155/94, respirations 22, temperature 37.8° C. On physical exam, he was diaphoretic with skin cool to the touch and no obvious bruises or abrasions. His lung sounds were clear, and he denied headache, vomiting, or shortness of breath.

Next, fill in the blanks in the patient data column using the above patient scenario. Under the Data Type heading, put an S for subjective data, or an O for objective data.

Patient Data		Data Type
Patient's age		S
Complaint of pain (Y/N)		S
Excessive gas and bloating (Y/N)		O
Dizziness (Y/N)		S
Pulse rate		O
Diaphoretic (Y/N)		O
Clear lung sounds (Y/N)		O
Shortness of breath (Y/N)		S
Vomiting (Y/N)		O
Nausea (Y/N)		S
Bruising (Y/N)		O
Elevated blood pressure (Y/N)		O

PART II: COMPONENTS OF THE NURSING PROCESS

Refer to the following scenario to answer the questions below:

A 69-year-old woman went to see her physician to get a renewal of her current medication prescriptions. She has a history of peptic ulcers and has been taking Pepcid for this problem. She has an allergy to morphine and adhesive tape. She has also been having increasing back pain and leg cramps for several weeks.

1. The chief complaint for this patient (or reason to see the physician) for this current visit is:
   1. peptic ulcers.
   2. back pain and leg cramps.
   3. renewal of medications.
   4. inability to tolerate Pepcid.

2. The physician asked the nurse to assist in obtaining vital signs on this patient. While taking her blood pressure, the nurse notices some areas of redness over her arm, which are reported to the physician. This important finding represents what type of assessment data?
   1. inspection
   2. palpation
   3. percussion
   4. auscultation

3. During the course of the visit to the physician, the patient tells the nurse she takes vitamins and herbal products to help her stomach. The best response to this would be to tell the patient: *(Select one answer.)*
   1. "I don't think the physician would like you to take those products."
   2. "I suspect your doctor would like to know that you are also taking those products."
   3. "I have tried those products also and recommend that you take them."
   4. "I think they are a waste of money."
   5. "I know that these products won't help your stomach."

   Explain why you chose the above answer.
   Because the nurse cannot assume what the doctor will say, and #2 is true that the info the patient shared the doctor would probably like to know

4. How does the LPN/LVN decide what to tell the patient about a medicine he or she is taking? *(Select all that apply.)*
   1. nursing care plan
   2. detailed history of the present illness
   3. six rights of medication administration
   4. provide simple answers to the patient's questions
   5. It is not the nurse's role to tell the patient anything.

5. Give some examples of things the nurse might tell the patient in answer to the following questions:
   1. "I don't feel like swallowing the pill now. Could you just leave it on my bedside table and I'll take it later?"
   2. "What is that blue pill for?"
   3. "I have a headache. Could my new medicine have caused it?"
   4. "I took my new antibiotic an hour ago. Now I feel itchy all over, my tongue is swelling, and I am having trouble breathing. Is this normal?"

6. In implementing a drug order for a hospitalized patient, which of the following things might be done? *(Select all that apply.)*
   1. determine the last pain medication given
   2. give the correct dosage of the medication
   3. know the patient's family history
   4. get the patient to sit up to take the drug
   5. know why the medication is being given to the patient

PART III: NURSING DRUG HISTORY

1. When taking a patient's drug history, it is important that the nurse accurately find out about: *(Select all that apply.)*
   1. health care provider goals for patient treatment.
   2. whether the patient has diabetes and high blood pressure.
   3. all medications the patient may be taking, both prescription and over-the-counter.
   4. the adverse effect and the therapeutic effect of the drug.
   5. the last time the patient had a tetanus booster.
   6. the source of the information—primary, secondary, or tertiary.

2. Sources of information that the nurse uses to obtain a drug history include: primary (P), secondary (S), and tertiary (T). Indicate the following type of information using the correct letter.

Type of Information	Sources of Information
Other nurses	
Patient	
Family members	
Physician	
Laboratory values	
Internet database of medications	
Old medication records	
Pharmacology book	
Baby's mother	

3. Discuss with your classmates what you would do if the information the patient told you is different from what the health care provider has written in the chart. What would you do about it?

PART IV: PLANNING DRUG THERAPY

1. The nurse has been assigned to care for a 76-year-old woman who has pneumonia. The physician has ordered a broad-spectrum antibiotic, vancomycin, for her because she has a penicillin allergy. What teaching is important to cover in the plan for this patient? *(Select all that apply.)*
   1. what effect the antibiotic will have
   2. what adverse drug effects to watch for
   3. any drug allergies that the patient has
   4. the route the medication will be given
   5. how long to expect to be taking the drug

2. Antibiotics especially need to be given on time if they are to help the patient get well. What test might be ordered to see if the antibiotic is working?
   1. a gallbladder x-ray
   2. clotting time measured
   3. specimens for culture
   4. thyroid function studies

3. When giving drugs to patients, the nurse's responsibility includes checking for which two types of responses to drug therapy?
   1. adverse effects and side effects
   2. therapeutic effects and adverse effects
   3. therapeutic effects and common responses
   4. adverse effects and allergic reactions

4. If a patient develops itching and shortness of breath and faints after taking a drug, he or she is probably having a/an _____.
   The nurse's response would be to _____
   _____.

PART V: THE DRUG ORDER

1. The nurse has received an order to begin Lasix (furosemide) 40 mg daily. What information is missing from the order that the nurse needs prior to medication administration? *(Select all that apply.)*
   1. date medication was ordered
   2. name of the medication
   3. dosage of the medication
   4. time the medication is to be given
   5. route of administration

2. Look up information about Penicillin VK and then consider the following drug order: Penicillin 5 mg twice a day. *(Select all that apply.)*
   1. The drug dosage is invalid.
   2. The drug should be given four times a day.
   3. The medication can be given as ordered only to pediatric patients.
   4. The order does not have a proper route identified.

3. What would the nurse do if he or she had received the order in #2?
   1. Give the drug as ordered.
   2. Give the drug once and call the physician about when to give it again.
   3. Give the drug by mouth as that is the usual way to give penicillin.
   4. Hold the drug and seek further information within the hour.

PART VI: MASTERING CHAPTER CONCEPTS

1. Discuss with your classmates what you would do if you believe you have been given an order for a medication that does not seem correct. How would you handle it?

2. What kind of resources are available to you to learn about the medications that you are going to be studying?

3. What is the difference between your pharmacology textbook and a drug reference book?

4. Go to the Internet and look up the drug hydro-chlorothiazide. Find at least six different web-sites that give you information about this drug. Talk with your classmates about how you would determine which Internet sites might have the most reliable information. Is there a difference in the quality of information that comes from a website that ends in *.gov*, *.com*, or *.org*? Which site to be you believe might give the most accurate information?

5. Go to www.cdc.gov. What types of information can you find here?

6. Go to www.pfizer.com. What types of information can you find here?

7. Go to www.apa.org. What types of information can you find here?

8. Go to a search engine like Yahoo or Google. Search the name of a drug. What types of web-sites show up in your search? How do you compare these sites to the other sites you have been viewing?

Patient Teaching and Health Literacy

 Go to http://evolve.elsevier.com/edmunds/lpn/ for additional activities and exercises.

PART I: HELPING PATIENTS BECOME COMPLIANT

Reminder: There are two basic reasons why patients have difficulty following their treatment plans. Either they do not understand what they should do, or they understand what they should do but fail to do it. They may not believe that they need to carry out the treatment plan. If they do believe they should do something, they may fail to carry out the plan because they might not have the money, the time, or the ability to do it. Everyone who works with a patient should look for teaching opportunities. The nurse, in teaching the patient, must be able to answer questions, give information, and address patient concerns.

1. The nurse has been helping the patient select food on her hospital menu. The patient has recently been diagnosed with diabetes. She says that she can eat anything with the exception of sugar in her coffee. The nurse's best response is:
   1. "What did the RN tell you about eating and managing your diabetes?"
   2. "That will help you by not using sugar in your coffee."
   3. "What is your understanding of how diabetes affects you?"
   4. "I think you are playing games with me."

2. The nurse in the physician's office sees a teenage girl who is in college. She tells the nurse she is sick all the time. She says that she can't afford to buy fruits or vegetables because they cost so much money. She knows she should eat better, but she has to make choices about how she spends her money and would rather eat pizza than fruit. The nurse's best response is:
   1. "You should eat a better diet than pizza, which is not good for you. It will make you fat."
   2. "What about other foods that are nutritious and do not cost a lot of money?"
   3. "Ask your mother to send you the money for fruits and vegetables."
   4. "I would think that buying pizza gets expensive. Think more about your health."

3. Mrs. Maxwell, age 73, is prescribed digitalis in the morning, a beta blocker twice a day, a diuretic three times a day, ASA 82 mg every day, and calcium 1200 mg every evening. The nurse notices that Mrs. Maxwell has lots of medicine left over from the last time she filled her prescriptions, and realizes that the patient isn't taking her medicine as ordered. Mrs. Maxwell also seems a little confused. What might be the best way to handle this?
   1. Organize the medications alphabetically and tell her to take them according to a chart you made.
   2. Discuss each of the medications she is taking to determine her understanding of their purpose.
   3. Ask her why she doesn't take the medications like the doctor ordered.
   4. Explore with her any problems she may be having taking her medications.

PART II: COMMUNICATING WITH THE PATIENT (HEALTH LITERACY)

1. What are some barriers to learning that patients may have? *(Select all that apply.)*
    1. A language barrier exists between the nurse and the patient; the patient is from another country.
    2. The patient has limited ability to understand and read.
    3. The patient has an incomplete understanding of what will happen if he or she does not take the medications.
    4. The patient cannot read the patient education materials provided.

2. Research suggests that all of these things might make health-related materials difficult for patients to understand except:
    1. the language used to describe side effects is frightening to the patient.
    2. the material was never discussed with the patient, who remains unsure of some of the meanings of the words in the material.
    3. the patient has a health disparity, meaning he or she can't read.
    4. talking with patients to understand what they know about the medications they are taking.

3. What technique might interfere with patient learning?
    1. Use fear-arousing comments to scare the patient into compliance.
    2. Determine the patient's need to learn.
    3. Select the best teaching method to use.
    4. Determine the patient's willingness to learn.

4. The patient's prescription reads to take the medicine 3 times a day for 5 days. When the patient returns to the clinic feeling worse, the nurse discovers that he has been taking the medicine 5 times a day for 3 days. The nurse should:
    1. Tell him that he made a big mistake that made him sicker.
    2. Clarify the correct information and sympathize with him that it is easy to get mixed up.
    3. Tell him that it is the pharmacy's fault, as they should have explained this to him.
    4. Tell him that it really doesn't matter as he has just gotten his medicine faster than ordered.

Replace the underlined word with a simpler layman's term that would be easier for the patient to understand when giving the following instructions.

5. "When you wake up in the morning, take your <u>antiinfective</u> prior to eating your breakfast."
    1. antibiotic
    2. cholesterol medication
    3. kidney drug
    4. allergy medication

6. "One of the potential complications of this medicine is <u>nephrotoxicity</u>."
    1. an allergic reaction
    2. kidney failure
    3. heart disease
    4. an infection

7. "Drug interactions may cause adverse reactions. Notify your health care professional if you have any <u>hematologic symptoms</u>."
    1. severe itching and a rash
    2. any trouble breathing or shortness of breath
    3. fever and chills
    4. unexplained bleeding or bruising

8. Take turns with your classmates pretending to give a patient information on the following subjects:

    *   You will have to take this medicine for the rest of your life.
    *   The medicine is likely to cost a lot of money.
    *   There are side effects associated with this medicine.

    Evaluate the discussions you had. What things made giving the information the most helpful? Did you all agree on the best ways to explain things?

PART III: THE PROCESS OF PATIENT EDUCATION

Deciding What the Patient Needs to Know

1. What are the key points to review with the patient concerning his or her medications? *(Select all that apply.)*
   1. the reason for taking the medication
   2. the name of the drug
   3. any special instructions about when to take the drug and how often
   4. any side effects that are common
   5. to call the doctor if he or she misses a dose
   6. special precautions when taking the drug; for instance, to avoid sunlight

2. When might be the best opportunity to teach the patient?
   1. When he has just been told he has diabetes.
   2. When he is all ready to be discharged.
   3. When he asks a question about his medications or disease.
   4. Right after the physician has left so you can clarify the patient's understanding.

   Why do you believe the answer you chose was the best answer?

3. How would the nurse teach the patient who doesn't want to know the things the nurse wants to teach him?
   1. Tell the patient he will have to know it before he will be able to go home.
   2. Explain that the doctor expects him to take the medicine accurately.
   3. Explore the reasons the patient has for not wanting to learn right now.
   4. Hand him the written materials and tell him to read it later.

4. What statement by the patient will indicate that the patient has learned what the nurse is trying to teach?
   1. "I get it now."
   2. "My spouse will give me my medications."
   3. "When I get home, I will reread this material so I will know what to do."
   4. "I understand when to take my medications and the side effects to watch for."

5. What are some helpful tips for teaching patients effectively?
   1. Try to cover as much teaching information as possible every time the patient comes to the clinic.
   2. Have the patient read the information provided.
   3. Teaching is hard, so stick to using the teaching method that works best for you.
   4. Give praise and show support for a change in behavior.

6. The nurse is talking with a new patient in the clinic and the patient has just said, "I really am not sure what this drug is for." What is the nurse's best response?
   1. "I will tell you and then you must repeat it back to me."
   2. "Let me see the drug, I will tell you."
   3. "What do you remember about your medications?"
   4. "Let's go over your medications, I can help teach you some ways to remember them."

7. Discuss with your classmates why you sometimes fail to take a medicine (antibiotics, painkiller) that has been ordered. Why did you not take the medicine? How could someone help you change your behavior?

8. **Challenge activity:** Based on your reading, match the benefits and problems in using the following teaching methods. *(More than one answer may apply.)*

Teaching Method	Benefits and/or Problems
1. _____ Easy to give instructions	a. Verbal instructions
2. _____ Time-consuming method	b. Written materials
3. _____ Difficult to determine understanding	c. Audiovisual materials
4. _____ Best method for learning	d. Demonstrations
5. _____ Requires different teaching skills	e. Combinations of these methods

PART IV: MASTERING PATIENT TEACHING AND HEALTH LITERACY

1. Some patients will want to use the Internet to learn about their disease and the medications they are taking. What things can you tell or give patients to help them if they like to learn using the computer? What problems might these patients have when they rely on the computer for their information? How might you help them avoid these problems?

Legal Aspects Affecting the Administration of Medications

chapter

3

 Go to http://evolve.elsevier.com/edmunds/lpn/ for additional activities and exercises.

PART I: CLASSIFYING DRUGS

Major concept to understand: Drugs are classified according to their risk for abuse. Higher-risk drugs have special requirements for their handling and recording.

Challenge Activity: Using your textbook, look up the following medications and, based on the information provided, try to classify each medication according to whether you believe it might be a "CS" for controlled substance, "PD" for prescription drug, or may be purchased "OTC" for over the counter. Note: Some medications may have more than one classification, based on dosage.

1. _____ lorazepam (Ativan)
2. _____ captopril (Capoten)
3. _____ famotidine (Pepcid)
4. _____ clindamycin (Cleocin)
5. _____ raloxifene (Evista)
6. _____ diphenhydramine (Benadryl)
7. _____ fexofenadine (Allegra)
8. _____ levothyroxine (Levothroid)
9. _____ phenylephrine (Neo-Synephrine)
10. _____ docusate (Colace)
11. _____ guaifenesin (Robitussin-AC)
12. _____ albuterol (Ventolin)
13. _____ ibuprofen (Advil)

14. Why does it matter to you as an LPN/LVN what the drug classification might be?

PART II: IDENTIFYING PARTS OF THE PATIENT'S CHART

Major concept to understand: The chart provides information that may be useful to the nurse while he or she is giving medications to the patient.

Challenge Activity: Traditional sections of the patient's chart include the following.

a. Summary sheet
b. Graphic record
c. History and physical examination
d. Problem list
e. Progress notes
f. Laboratory tests
g. Consultations
h. Physician's orders

Indicate in which part or parts of the patient's chart you would look for the following information:

1. _____ Blood pressure
2. _____ Report from the cardiologist
3. _____ Bed rest with bathroom privileges
4. _____ Major diagnosis
5. _____ Weight
6. _____ Description of heart sounds
7. _____ Tetracycline 500 mg orally four times daily
8. _____ CT scan on Thursday
9. _____ Enema given
10. _____ Response to pain medication
11. _____ Intake and output record
12. _____ Electrolyte report
13. _____ CBC with differential on Thursday
14. _____ Occupation
15. _____ Insurance

16. Why would an LPN/LVN want to know this information about the chart if he or she is just going to administer medication?

PART III: MORE PRACTICE UNDERSTANDING MEDICATION ORDERS

Major concept to understand: All drug orders are not of the same importance.

Challenge Activity: *Explain the following drug orders. Classify the order as an "SO" for standing order, "stat" for stat order, "prn" for prn order, or "S" for single order.*

Classification

1. stat   Haldol 5 mg IM stat
2. prn   MOM 30 mL orally prn constipation
3. prn   Trazodone 150 mg orally prn insomnia
4. SO   Lanoxin 0.25 mg orally every morning
5. SO   Dilantin 100 mg orally three times daily
6. S   Ancef 1 g IV piggyback on call to OR
7. SO   Metamucil l package in 8 oz of cold water every morning before breakfast
8. prn   Ventolin inhaler ii puffs prn wheezing
9. SO   Prednisone 10 mg daily orally x 7 days
10. stat   Lasix 20 mg IV now
11. SO   Aspirin 325 mg orally every morning
12. prn   Tigan 200 mg suppository rectally every 6 hours if nauseated

13. The patient is on his way back from surgery. The patient is in extreme pain, but has been given morphine. Morphine has caused the patient to vomit, so the surgeon orders medication for nausea. Think about the problem this patient is having. Would this prescription order likely be a stat order or a prn order?

PART IV: LEGAL ASPECTS SURROUNDING THE ADMINISTRATION OF MEDICATIONS

Major concept to understand: Compared to other physician orders, using the nursing process and following all the rules are especially important when giving medications.

1. The charge nurse is getting ready to leave the hospital unit after a 12-hour shift. The nurse just coming on duty meets the charge nurse at the locked narcotic box to complete the inventory count required at the end of each shift. During the count, it is discovered that a 10-mg ampule of morphine is missing. What will they do next? *(Select all that apply.)*
   1. Check with other nurses to determine who removed morphine from the cabinet during the shift.
   2. Check charts of patients receiving morphine to see if someone gave the medicine but didn't sign for it.
   3. Count the inventory again, there must be some mistake.
   4. Notify the nursing supervisor and fill out an incident report. (patient report)
   5. It is only one ampule so it isn't a big deal.
   6. Check the garbage to see if there is a broken ampule there.

2. Do you have any other ideas about what might have happened in this situation? Depending upon your answers, what are the different ways you might proceed?

   interview nurses (interrogate)

3. One of the doctors asks the nurse if he can borrow the key to the narcotics box because he needs to give a patient some medicine before she leaves for a procedure. The nurse should:
   1. give him the key but make sure he signs out the narcotic on the sign-out sheet.
   2. open the narcotics box for him and give him the medicine, but do not give him the key.
   3. call the nursing supervisor because the doctor should never be given narcotics.
   4. tell the doctor that if he will write the order, you will be happy to give the patient the narcotic.

4. What is the difference between controlled substances and prescription drugs?
   1. All drugs sold in drugstores are controlled over-the-counter drugs.
   2. The Food and Drug Administration considers all medications to be controlled substances.
   3. Controlled substances have a greater potential for abuse.
   4. Controlled substances are not available through prescriptions.

5. A wide variety of medications are available over the counter (OTC). Patients often do not report to their health care provider that they are taking these products. Why might this be a problem?
   1. Because OTC products could be addictive.
   2. Because some OTC products may cause problems when taken with other prescription drugs that may be ordered.
   3. Because the patient taking two different types of drugs could then become dependent on the prescription drugs.
   4. It would not be a problem because OTC products are of a very low dosage.

6. The nurse was hurrying to give the patient her medication and did not read the medication card carefully. She gave the patient 2500 mg of tetracycline instead of 250 mg. She should:
   1. tell the patient immediately what has happened.
   2. discuss the problem with the head nurse and physician to determine what to do.
   3. call the pharmacy to see if they think there will be a problem.
   4. check the patient's vital signs to make certain he or she is still breathing.

PART V: ETHICAL SITUATIONS

Major concept to understand: Often the best thing to do is not the easiest thing to do.

1. The nurse sees a coworker secretly slip some medications into her pocket. What should the nurse do next?
   1. Tell the charge nurse what you witnessed.
   2. Ask the coworker what medications she has in her pocket.
   3. Ignore the incident, it is not your business.
   4. Tell the nurse on the next shift about the coworker's actions.

2. The nurse has been at work for 5 hours and has a terrible headache. Two hours ago, the nurse took some ibuprofen she brought from home and it did not help. There are some pain pills left over from a patient who died that are still in the cabinet. Should the nurse take one of these pills for her headache?
   1. Yes, the drugs will probably just be thrown away.
   2. No, the drugs have to be returned to the pharmacy.
   3. Yes, in this situation, the drugs are for anybody who wants them.
   4. No, the drugs will be sent to the patient's family.

3. The nurses' station is very busy and there are lots of new admissions. It is 3 PM and the medication nurses realize that they forgot to pass the 1 PM medications to one patient. The drug was an antibiotic. What should the nurse do next?
   1. Give the medication late and do not tell anyone.
   2. Give the medication late and tell the pharmacist and the next nurse.
   3. Give the medication late and tell the charge nurse and the doctor and fill out an incident report.
   4. Do not give the medication, but report the omission immediately to the charge nurse and find out if it should be given late.

4. The patient is disoriented and restless. When the nurse approaches her to give her the medication cup, she knocks the pills on the floor. The next delivery from the pharmacy will not be on that shift. What should the nurse do after the pills are picked up off the floor?
   1. Give the pills to the patient.
   2. Throw the pills away.
   3. Skip the dose and document in the patient's chart.
   4. Report the incident to your head nurse or team leader and order more medications.

Foundations and Principles of Pharmacology

Go to http://evolve.elsevier.com/edmunds/lpn/ for additional activities and exercises.

PART I: PHARMACOLOGIC DEFINITIONS AND DRUG NAMES

1. Pharmacokinetics is:
   1. the use of drugs to treat an illness.
   2. the action drugs have on your body.
   3. how the body reacts to the drugs you take.
   4. a confusing term that just means medications.

2. The doctor has ordered the following drugs for the patient: promethazine, spironolactone, and lisinopril. These names represent which type of drug name?
   1. trade names
   2. generic names
   3. chemical names
   4. official names

3. When a drug is described as an *agonist*, it means it:
   1. can only work by absorption.
   2. will be effective against bacteria.
   3. produces an action similar to the body's own chemicals.
   4. stops other chemicals from working in the body.

Use your textbook to look up the following drugs to answer questions 4 and 5.

4. Use a "C" for chemical names, "T" for trade names, and "G" for generic names for the following medications:
   1. _____ meperidine
   2. _____ Lanoxin
   3. _____ Zovirax
   4. _____ ribavirin
   5. _____ loratadine

5. Match the following generic drug names with their trade names:

1. _____ acetylsalicylic acid	a.	Valium
2. _____ chlorothiazide	b.	Diuril
3. _____ diazepam	c.	Aspirin
4. _____ ethacrynic acid	d.	Ultram
5. _____ tramadol	e.	Edecrin

6. Drugs that act on a receptor in the body to stop a reaction are referred to as:
   1. agonists.
   2. partial agonists.
   3. antagonists.
   4. antireceptors.

7. Why does it matter which drug name is used?

8. The patient in the hospital is taking chlorothiazide and Lanoxin. The patient says that at home she takes Diuril. Should the nurse call the physician for an order for the other drug?

PART II: IDENTIFYING DRUG PROCESSES

Major concept to understand: Medicines must be absorbed, distributed, metabolized, and excreted.

Absorption

1. The patient tells the nurse that he always just swallows his medications dry because it really doesn't matter if he swallows with water; the drugs still work the same. What is the nurse's best response?
   1. "The drugs actually absorb into your system faster when you take them with water, which will allow them to dissolve."
   2. "The drugs need to be taken with water so that you will not choke on them."
   3. "The drugs work the same with or without water. You are right, it makes no difference."
   4. "The drugs will need to be dissolved before they can be diffused throughout your body, so you must take water with them."

2. Identify the route of administration for the following examples by using "E" for enteral, "P" for parenteral, and "Q" for percutaneous.

   _____ inhaler medications

   _____ topical medications

   _____ intravenous medications

   _____ rectal suppositories

   _____ sublingual (under the tongue)

   _____ oral medications

   _____ intramuscular medications

3. The rate of absorption depends on which of the following processes? *(Select all that apply.)*
   1. the amount of blood flow through the tissues
   2. the type of medication (antibiotic, calcium channel blocker, ACE inhibitor, etc.)
   3. the route of administration of the medication
   4. the way the drug dissolves in solution

4. From the following pairs of medications indicate (with an X) which one of the two you would anticipate to have the desired effect faster if they had been given at the same time.

Proventil bronchodilator aerosol		*or*		Compazine rectal suppository
Adrenalin in oil SQ		*or*		Aqueous adrenalin SQ
Nitroglycerin SL		*or*		Metamucil 1 glass
Toradol IV		*or*		Vasotec oral
Enteric-coated aspirin		*or*		Haldol IM

Distribution

5. Medications that are able to cross the placental barrier are said to be:
   1. evenly distributed.
   2. distributed throughout all types of tissues equally.
   3. able to affect the fetus.
   4. unable to cross the blood-brain barrier.

Metabolism

6. Nurses need to understand how medications are handled by the body for the following reasons. *(Select all that apply.)*
   1. It is important to teach patients the reason for the different routes of administration.
   2. To know when to expect the drugs to be the strongest and when their action will be over.
   3. To know when the patient will need to go to the bathroom.
   4. The cytochrome P-450 system might reduce or increase the effectiveness of some drugs.

7. Patients who have liver disease are at risk for drug intoxication or overdose because:
   1. the liver usually inactivates drugs.
   2. the kidneys usually inactivate drugs.
   3. only medications that are taken orally will cause this.
   4. the GI tract usually inactivates drugs.

Excretion

8. It is important for nurses to be aware of their patients' urine output and normal bowel habits because:
    1. liver and kidneys are the main organs that remove drugs from the body.
    2. kidneys and GI tract are the main organs that remove drugs from the body.
    3. skin and the lungs are the main organs that remove drugs from the body.
    4. lungs and the liver are the main organs that remove drugs from the body.

9. What does the phrase *drug half-life of 30 to 60 minutes* mean?
    1. It means that the nurse should give the drug every 30 to 60 minutes.
    2. It means that the drug is only half as effective after 60 minutes.
    3. It describes how long it takes the drug to be absorbed.
    4. It describes how long it takes the body to remove 50% of the drug from the body.

10. An elderly female patient has depression. She is started on a product that takes 3 to 4 weeks to work. After about 2 weeks, the patient becomes very nervous and agitated. The doctor tells her that this is from the medication and that the drug has a long half-life. The patient doesn't understand what this means and asks the nurse to explain it. What should the nurse say?

PART III: CLASSIFYING TYPES OF DRUG REACTIONS

Major concept to understand: Giving drugs is not like following a recipe because patients often respond differently to the same drug. It is essential that the nurse help watch how the drug affects the patient.

Read the following scenario:

Ms. Carmen, a 48-year-old patient, was admitted to the hospital with pneumonia. She has an elevated temperature, chills, and a cough that has produced a large amount of green-colored sputum. She also reports severe congestion and a sore throat. Ms. Carmen has had high blood pressure for several years and takes propranolol daily to reduce it. For the pneumonia, the patient was started on therapy consisting of ciprofloxacin 500 mg IVPB every 6

hours, Tylenol 650 mg every 4 hours prn for temperature elevation, and Robitussin cough syrup, 30 mL every 4 hours prn.

The following is a list of possible symptoms that are an effect of all the medications the patient is taking. Decide which ones are expected effects "E," side effects "S," adverse effects "A," or allergic reactions "R," and place the correct letter corresponding to the patient response.

1. _____ temperature reduced from 38.5° C to 37.2° C
2. _____ skin rash
3. _____ cough suppressed
4. _____ sputum changes color from green to yellow
5. _____ blood pressure drops from 140/85 to 110/72
6. _____ pain reduced
7. _____ white blood cell count increases
8. _____ nausea
9. _____ short of breath and feeling of impending doom
10. _____ drowsiness
11. _____ hepatotoxicity (liver damage)
12. _____ nasal congestion

PART IV: RECOGNIZING TYPES OF DRUG INTERACTIONS

1. While discussing the patient's medications, he tells the nurse that he is allergic to morphine. The nurse asks him to explain what happens when he takes morphine. Which of the following answers to this question indicates a true allergy?
    1. "I get nauseated when I take morphine."
    2. "I get lightheaded when I take morphine."
    3. "I get a rash when I take morphine."
    4. "I smell a funny odor when I take morphine."

2. The patient is taking phenytoin (Dilantin) for seizures and has started to develop the following symptoms: drowsiness, poor memory, slurred speech, and poor coordination. These represent:
    1. an allergic reaction.
    2. a drug interaction.
    3. an adverse reaction.
    4. a normal side effect.

3. The patient says "The doctor told me that I am allergic to penicillin. Does that mean I cannot take any antibiotics ever again? The nurse's response would be:
    1. "It means you can never take any antibiotics again, and you need to wear a Medic-alert bracelet."
    2. "It means that you will have to remember to tell your doctor every time you are prescribed any antibiotics so that we can avoid using any penicillin-type drugs."
    3. "It means that you will have a severe anaphylactic reaction and die the next time you take any penicillin."
    4. "It means that you will always react to penicillin with an idiosyncratic response and must tell your doctor."

4. Give an example of each of the following phrases:
    1. anaphylactic reaction:

    2. side effect:

    3. idiosyncratic response:

    4. hypersensitivity response:

    If you don't know what the phrase *idiosyncratic response* means, look it up and give some examples of this type of response.

5. The patient was taking metoprolol for hypertension and his blood pressure became elevated. This indicates what type of possible reaction?
    1. an anaphylactic reaction
    2. an idiosyncratic response
    3. a hypersensitivity reaction
    4. a normal side effect

Lifespan and Cultural Modifications

Go to http://evolve.elsevier.com/edmunds/lpn/ for additional activities and exercises.

PART I: SPECIAL CONSIDERATIONS IN THE PEDIATRIC, GERIATRIC, AND PREGNANT OR BREASTFEEDING PATIENT

Major concept to understand: Special attention must be paid when giving medications to children, older adults, and pregnant or breastfeeding women so that drug use is effective and not harmful.

1. A 34-year-old mother came into the clinic with her 4-year-old child, who was being treated for an ear infection. She asked the nurse "Does it matter if I give my child over-the-counter medications? They are safe for children aren't they?" The nurse's best response would be:
   1. "Yes, all over-the-counter medications are safe to give children, because they have been tested."
   2. "It is important to read the label on any medication that you get over the counter to see if it is safe."
   3. "Children who have ear infections need to take only prescribed medications."
   4. "Over-the-counter medications are safe for adults but not for children."

2. The nurse is reviewing an order for two children ages 2 years and 12 years. She notices that the amounts are the same for both children for the same medication. The nurse knows that medications for children:
   1. are metabolized differently depending on the age of the child, so the order needs to be questioned.
   2. are weight-based, so the children must be the same weight, so the order is correct.
   3. are only effective within a narrow range, so the order is correct.
   4. always have higher doses for younger children, so the order needs to be questioned.

3. Fill in the blanks. Physiologic processes that affect how neonates metabolize drugs are:
   1. _____ gastric acid.
   2. _____ body water volume.
   3. _____ body mass.
   4. _____ liver.

4. The nurse understands which of the following is accurate regarding injections for children?
   1. Giving an injection to an infant is preferred to other routes of administration.
   2. Increased blood supply to muscles leads to more drug being absorbed.
   3. The vastus lateralis muscle has a more rapid absorption rate compared to the deltoid muscle.
   4. Absorption rates for injections do not vary as all muscles have the same blood flow.

5. A 78-year-old man has diabetes, hypertension, and arthritis and takes many medications. Because he is older, what gradual changes in his body might affect the medications he takes? *(Select all that apply.)*
   1. Reduced gastric emptying and decreased bowel motility reduces drug excretion.
   2. The GI tract will have less acid and affect the body's ability to absorb the drugs.
   3. The liver function slows down, resulting in more of the drug staying in the blood.
   4. Protein-bound drugs circulate freely when albumin levels are decreased.

6. Two 65-year-old men taking the same antihypertensive medication come into the clinic. One of them is very overweight and in poor physical condition, and the other patient is a very large man who plays tennis and swims every day. What one factor places the overweight patient at higher risk for drug toxicities than the patient in good physical condition?
   1. An overweight person requires less medication than a normal-weight person.
   2. An overweight person requires the same amount of medication as a normal-weight person.
   3. An overweight person requires more medication than a normal-weight person.
   4. An overweight person requires more medication because they develop tolerance more easily than a normal-weight person.

7. An older woman is diagnosed with diabetes and started on insulin therapy. She has very poor vision and her hands are swollen with arthritis, making self-administration of insulin difficult. What suggestions might the nurse consider in helping her to take her medications? *(Select all that apply.)*
   1. Suggest that if she loses weight she probably won't need to take insulin.
   2. Suggest she use a magnifying glass when filling her syringe.
   3. Suggest that she move into a nursing home because she cannot take care of herself anymore.
   4. Explore options about family members who may be available to help her.

8. Mrs. Liddle lives alone. She is on a fixed income and has a hard time buying her medications. The nurse discovers that she cuts her pills in half and sometimes skips doses to reduce costs. What are some ways the nurse can help with this problem?
   1. Remind her she will get sicker if she doesn't take them.
   2. Explore options with the doctor to see if she can skip some of her doses.
   3. Ask social services to there are ways to help with the financial cost of her medications.
   4. Do not interfere, as there is no solution to her problem.

9. Mrs. Kline discovers that she is pregnant. She is very upset because she has been taking an antibiotic for the last 2 weeks for a severe case of bronchitis. What should the nurse tell her?
   1. "Many drugs are contraindicated during pregnancy; you have put your unborn child at risk."
   2. "Don't worry; it is safe to take medications during pregnancy."
   3. "The medications you take during your pregnancy affect the genetics of your unborn child."
   4. "Certain antibiotics do produce birth defects (teratogenic). You need to consult with your physician about this."

10. Mrs. Partridge, age 74, takes many medications for arthritis. Her daughter is worried because her mother has new problems with disorientation and complains of a headache. The nurse discovers Mrs. Partridge is also having some mental function changes and is depressed. These signs and symptoms are indicative of:
    1. typical older adult behavior.
    2. nonadherence with her medication regimen.
    3. teratogenic effects of arthritis medications.
    4. possible adverse effects of medications.

11. It is important for the nurse to recognize medications that might be associated with producing birth defects (teratogenic). Put a checkmark next to the medications that fall into this category. *(Select all that apply.)*
    1. lithium _____
    2. alcohol _____
    3. caffeine _____
    4. anticonvulsants _____
    5. warfarin _____
    6. anticancer agents _____
    7. vitamins _____
    8. tetracycline _____

12. Special concerns for most older adult patients taking medications include:
    1. poor memory of older persons.
    2. chronic use of over-the-counter medications.
    3. drugs are processed more slowly in older adults.
    4. nonadherence issues with all medications.

13. Aging affects the absorption of drugs and the older adult patient must be observed for which of the following body functions?
    1. Observe urine output for kidney function.
    2. Check physical activity level for mobility.
    3. Assess orientation for memory function.
    4. Observe for visual disturbances.

14. Missy Rockwood has a 3-week-old baby. She has developed severe mastitis in her right breast, and the doctor started her on a course of antibiotics for treatment. What should she do about breastfeeding?
    1. Switch to bottle-feeding while taking medication and express but discard her milk; resume breastfeeding when the infection is gone.
    2. Reassure her she can continue to breastfeed as this is the best nutrition for her baby.
    3. Switch to bottle-feeding while taking medications and express her milk but save it for later use; resume breastfeeding when the infection is gone.
    4. Continue breastfeeding as antibiotics will not pass into the breast milk.

15. The effects of aging on the kidney that might affect medication dosage include:
    1. an increase in creatinine excretion.
    2. the ability to remove more sodium.
    3. problems leading to water retention.
    4. a decrease in blood flow to the kidneys.

PART II: PRODUCTS USED THROUGHOUT THE LIFESPAN

Major concept to understand: Many patients, even when they are not sick, will take medications throughout their lives for different reasons. Patients take these medications with little supervision or education from nurses.

Challenge Activity: Match the benefits or goals of therapy with the correct category.

Medication Categories		Goals of Therapy
1. _____ immunizations	a.	increase male potency
2. _____ antidiabetic agents	b.	reduce risk for cardiovascular problems
3. _____ hormone replacement therapy	c.	decrease the risk for lung cancer
4. _____ cholesterol-lowering agents	d.	used along with exercise to increase weight loss
5. _____ smoking cessation	e.	improve chemical imbalances in the brain
6. _____ obesity drugs	f.	improve management of blood sugar
7. _____ contraception	g.	protect against communicable disease
8. _____ antidepressants	h.	reduce hot flashes
9. _____ drugs for impotence	i.	reduce risk for stroke
10. _____ aspirin	j.	reduce birth rate

PART III: CULTURAL INFLUENCES RELATED TO MEDICATIONS

Major concept to understand: What is culturally familiar and acceptable for patients may be important in helping them get well. When you encounter beliefs you don't understand, attempt to get more information.

1. A Hispanic patient came into the clinic newly diagnosed as having diabetes. The following concerns need to be addressed in teaching about the management of diabetes. *(Select all that apply.)*
   1. Use an interpreter as needed for any language barrier.
   2. Determine the extent of the patient's understanding about diabetes.
   3. Discuss values and beliefs regarding health care.
   4. Distribute pamphlets on diabetes and ask if there are any questions.

2. You are caring for a Hmong family who has a very ill child. Some important considerations while working with this family include:
   1. tell the family what should be done for their child.
   2. learn about the culture and respect the beliefs they have.
   3. tell the parents not to bring food to feed the child.
   4. allow the family to give their child traditional medicine they have brought from home.

3. Some medications cause a loss of appetite. What would be the best way to get someone from another culture to eat? *(Select all that apply.)*
   1. Explain to the patient that it is necessary to eat even if her appetite is gone.
   2. Force-feed her, as proper nutrition is key to getting better.
   3. Explore options that would allow a choice of food to eat.
   4. Offer options that may stimulate appetite, keeping the food appealing.

4. In teaching a patient about his thyroid replacement medication, it becomes clear that the patient feels very uncomfortable about taking medicine. He says he worries about being "addicted" to the medicine. How would you deal with this?
   1. Seek support from another nurse and insist the patient take his medications.
   2. Listen without judging to the patient's fears.
   3. Laugh and tell him he can't be addicted to this medicine.
   4. Ignore the concerns of the patient and consult the physician about this noncompliance.

5. A father has been drinking heavily, and when he comes to see his child in the hospital, he is clearly intoxicated. What should the nurse do about this situation?
   1. Pull the father aside and tell him that he is welcome to visit but should come back when he is sober.
   2. Ignore the situation. You have no business interfering.
   3. Alert security and have him removed from the hospital.
   4. Call the charge nurse and ask what to do.

6. When you enter the hospital room of a dying Native American, you find the patient's family is singing and has thrown dirt all over him. How should the nurse handle this situation?
   1. Brush off all the dirt and state that this is not proper to do in the hospital no matter what they believe.
   2. Call the charge nurse and ask what to do.
   3. Be respectful and ask the family to tell you what significance this has.
   4. Ask the family to leave so you can quickly hide this situation before doctor's rounds.

7. Mrs. Chen's husband has been very ill. When she visits him in the hospital, she is concerned that he is not getting better. The nurse finds that the wife has brought him some herbal tea to help him to "raise the hot element" in his body and "achieve balance." The nurse does not know what is in the tea. What would the nurse do?
   1. Throw the tea out and state that patients are only to have approved foods.
   2. Ask what the tea has in it and allow the use of this remedy, if it is determined to be safe.
   3. Call the charge nurse in and have the doctor paged about this situation.
   4. Explain that balance can only be achieved by following doctor's orders.

PART IV: STRATEGIES TO INCREASE PATIENT SUCCESS WITH DRUG TREATMENT

1. The patient is telling the nurse that he looked up his diagnosis online and discovered that the treatment the doctor wants to give him is one that is controversial. What are some appropriate responses? *(Select all that apply.)*
   1. "I worry that online information may not be from reliable sources."
   2. "I think you should discuss your concerns with your doctor."
   3. "I think that your doctor knows best and that you really should not question him."
   4. "I think that it is important to learn as much as you can about your illness."

2. Some consequences of drug nonadherence include:
   1. decreased health care costs because fewer drugs are taken.
   2. poor outcomes of treatment plans.
   3. decreased rates of outpatient services.
   4. more successful lawsuits.

3. ***Challenge Activity:*** *Match the underlying behavior with the situation in which drug noncompliance or nonadherence happens. Some answers may apply to more than one situation.*

Situation in which drug nonadherence occurs

1. _____ Medications are too expensive to take
2. _____ Does not like taking medications
3. _____ Lack of understanding about proper dose
4. _____ Poor understanding of how to store medications
5. _____ Intolerance to medications
6. _____ Busy lifestyle
7. _____ Can't remember to take medications on time

Factor underlying noncompliant behavior

a. Young child spits out medication every day
b. Woman fails to take her calcium replacement
c. Patient forgets daily dose of thyroid supplement
d. Patient forgets to take antihypertensive medication four times a day
e. Patient uses less nicotine replacement gum than ordered
f. Nitroglycerine was outdated and carried loosely with other cardiac medications in a box
g. Patient has diarrhea from medication

PART V: INTEGRATED CASE STUDY

Major concept to understand: You can't make patients take medications. By learning to understand patients, you may help them decide to take the medications and know how to do it properly.

As a public health nurse, you are sent to the home of Mr. Shen, an older Chinese man who has tuberculosis. He lives with many family members in a small apartment in the inner city. Several of his family members have developed positive PPD reactions since his diagnosis and are to take prophylactic (preventive) INH medications. Your community now has many drug-resistant strains of TB, and you are concerned about Mr. Shen's response to treatment. You have worked primarily with Hispanic and African-American patients and know nothing about Mr. Shen's culture.

1. What are some considerations that are important to keep in mind when the nurse is dealing with this family? *(Select all that apply.)*
    1. People of this culture are always difficult to deal with.
    2. Family situations require a different treatment plan so everyone is involved in the process.
    3. Noncompliance is common when there is poor understanding of the instructions.
    4. Cultural considerations are important to keep in mind and may affect what the patient is taught.

2. What are some ways to promote adherence to drug orders with this family?
    1. Learn about the culture and their beliefs regarding health care.
    2. Discuss the reason for taking the medications as prescribed with the father, who is the most important family member in this culture.
    3. Mail medication information to the house and expect them to read it.
    4. Tell the family that they are at risk of getting TB if they don't make the patient take the medicines.

3. Which factors listed below might make it difficult for patients to take their medicine as ordered? *(Select all that apply.)*
    1. medical mistakes
    2. ethnic background
    3. socioeconomic class
    4. education level
    5. family situation
    6. transportation issues

4. Health care workers can influence the patient relationship with the health care system by the following action.
    1. being friendly but firm in insisting on following directions
    2. writing down the patient complaints
    3. giving the family a copy of the plan of care
    4. taking time to motivate and encourage the patient
    5. expecting the patient to understand all instructions the first time

PART VI: MASTERING LIFESPAN AND CULTURAL CONCEPTS

1. With your classmates, make a list of several different cultures that are common in your community. If classmates have a way to talk with patients in these cultures, have them talk with several members of the cultures about their health beliefs. Alternatively, divide up the list and go to the Internet and try to find at least five things that the culture you are researching believes about health or disease. Share this information with your classmates. Discuss how this information might change how you talk to or deal with patients from these cultures.

2. If you have classmates from different cultures, perhaps they would be willing to share some of their experiences with being sick, having a baby, taking natural herbal products, or if their culture has beliefs that might make them less willing to take medicine. Ask them how you as the nurse can show respect for the patient's culture. What are the best ways to ask the patient about cultural beliefs?

3. What is ageism? As a group, discuss how you can change your behavior as a nurse to show your older patients that you are respectful of them.

Self-Care: Over-the-Counter Products, Herbal Therapies, and Drugs for Health Promotion

chapter

6

 Go to http://evolve.elsevier.com/edmunds/lpn/ for additional activities and exercises.

PART I: OVER-THE-COUNTER DRUG USAGE

Major concept to understand: Many patients take over-the-counter products that they may not realize could hurt them if not used carefully.

1. Patients learn information about over-the-counter (OTC) drugs from a variety of sources. The most accurate information will be from:
    1. magazines and the Internet.
    2. friends and relatives.
    3. advertisements on TV.
    4. their doctor.

2. Why do nurses need to be aware of which OTC medications their patients are taking?
    1. OTC medications are taking money away from the prescribed medications they should be buying.
    2. OTC medications are more likely to be taken than prescribed ones.
    3. OTC medications sometimes interfere with the effect of prescribed medications.
    4. OTC medications are unapproved home remedies.

3. What are some of the reasons patients take OTC medications? *(Select all that apply.)*
    1. They have tried other treatments without success.
    2. They have been told by other people that the OTC drug works.
    3. It is easier to read the information about OTC drugs than prescription medications.
    4. They find that it is cheaper to take OTC drugs than prescription medications.

4. Some of the OTC products that seem safe but might actually be harmful to pediatric or geriatric patients include:
    1. antihistamines for children because it is easy to overdose children.
    2. toothpastes for geriatric patients because they may swallow the compounds.
    3. sleep aids for children because they may contain aspirin, which is contraindicated in pediatric patients.
    4. antacids for geriatric patients because they may contain high levels of sodium.

5. What are the four ways OTC products differ from prescription medications?
    1. labeling information, greater availability, safer, more advertising, cheaper
    2. labeling information, safer, more advertising, more active ingredients
    3. labeling information, more advertising, more active ingredients, greater availability
    4. labeling information, more active ingredients, greater availability, safer, cheaper

6. What are the most common ailments for which patients use OTC medications?
    1. nasal congestion, smoking cessation, constipation, high blood pressure
    2. smoking cessation, constipation, peptic ulcer disorders, colds
    3. colds, constipation, vaginal infections, diverticulitis
    4. constipation, headaches, colds, diabetes

7. What are important teaching considerations to remember to discuss with patients regarding OTC product use?
   1. You often have to guess the amount of medication to give a child.
   2. Keep old OTC medications because they do not expire.
   3. If you have questions about the products, ask the doctor as the pharmacist doesn't know.
   4. If you think you are sick, read the label to help you decide if you need the product.
   5. If there is no improvement in symptoms, seek the advice of a health care provider.

8. Sarah Burton is a single mother who has an infant and a 4-year-old toddler who both have temperatures from a bad cold. She goes to the pharmacy to buy something cheap that she can give to both children. What concerns might you have about her doing this?
   1. The dosage will be different for the children because of their different weight.
   2. The infant will need to suck the medicine from a bottle while the other child should swallow a pill.
   3. The cheapest product isn't as effective as the more expensive brand name.
   4. Most products for colds are the same and are good for adults or children.

9. Your friend, Carl Dansbury, 53 years old, has been having heartburn at night when he goes to sleep. The doctor gave him a prescription for an expensive medication to take every day. Carl wants to buy something cheaper over the counter. You might tell him:
   1. he really doesn't need any medicine at all—just eat less and eat dinner earlier before he goes to bed.
   2. there are now lots of good, cheap OTC drugs for heartburn.
   3. almost all drugs for stomach problems are now OTC because they are so safe.
   4. because he takes other drugs for high blood pressure, he should probably buy what the doctor ordered.

PART II: ALTERNATIVE OR COMPLEMENTARY THERAPIES AND NUTRITIONAL SUPPLEMENTS

Major concept to understand: Many times there is little scientific knowledge about whether complementary or alternative therapies are helpful or harmful.

1. Alternative therapy and complementary therapy differ because:
   1. complementary therapy includes alternative therapy plus standard care.
   2. alternative therapy includes complementary therapy plus standard care.
   3. complementary therapy includes standard care but not alternative therapy.
   4. alternative therapy includes standard care but not complementary therapy.

2. Alternative therapy includes all except which of the following? *(Select all that apply.)*
   1. standard medical care
   2. aromatherapy
   3. chiropractic services
   4. acupuncture
   5. therapeutic touch
   6. herbal therapy

3. Which of the following is not a potential problem patients may face when using alternative therapy?
   1. no reliable information about the therapy
   2. little scientific testing has been done on the therapy
   3. herbal therapies are unregulated
   4. therapy is often very expensive

4. Some of the reasons patients are seeking alternative therapies and herbal therapies in particular are: *(Select all that apply.)*
   1. the desire to prevent disease.
   2. a distrust of their primary physician.
   3. for improving health.
   4. these are natural products and good for you.
   5. treating an existing illness for which standard therapy may not have been effective.
   6. finding an inexpensive substitute for standard care.

5. It is important for nurses to recognize that even though their patients may be seeing a physician, they could still be taking herbal remedies. What should be kept in mind when asking patients about their use of alternative therapies?
   1. Not all herbal remedies are approved by the FDA.
   2. Physicians will rarely be concerned about what patients take as long as they take their prescriptions.
   3. Serious medical problems may be worsened by the use of these remedies.
   4. Labels of supplements and herbal remedies can claim to cure or prevent cancer.

6. The nurse is taking care of a patient who insists that aromatherapy works. What does the nurse understand about this form of alternative medicine?
   1. Aromatherapy is endorsed by the medical community.
   2. Aromatherapy involves inhaling vapors from oils.
   3. Aromatherapy is harmless.
   4. Aromatherapy has much research backing up its claims.

7. When is it most likely that vitamins or minerals might be prescribed as a therapeutic regimen?
   1. cancer prevention
   2. to increase the overall sense of well-being
   3. to cope with stress
   4. to correct a deficiency

8. What is the difference between a natural vitamin and a synthetic one?
   1. Natural vitamins always contain some impurities.
   2. Synthetic vitamins may be less effective.
   3. Natural vitamins are cheaper.
   4. There is probably no difference. A vitamin is a vitamin.

9. How do antioxidants help to reduce the incidence of atherosclerosis or cancer?
   1. They speed up or increase LDL cholesterol oxidation.
   2. They slow down the process that causes some cells to become cancerous.
   3. They prevent the formation of plaque in blood vessels.
   4. They cause large amounts of vitamins to build up in the tissues.

10. What are some ways nurses can teach patients to maintain their health?
    1. Switch from smoking cigarettes to cigars.
    2. Take extra vitamins and minerals daily.
    3. Eat more fruits and vegetables.
    4. Exercise at least 2 hours daily.

PART III: INTEGRATED CASE STUDY

1. Jeannie Boyer and her husband are excited about having a baby. The nurse-midwife recommends taking folic acid. Jeannie is afraid any medication might hurt the fetus when she gets pregnant. What would the nurse tell Jeannie about folic acid and the risk to the fetus?

Fill in the blanks.

   1. Adequate amounts of folic acid before conception _____.

   2. Folic acid does not have to be in pill form; you can _____.

   3. Folic acid helps prevent _____, which result in spina bifida and anencephaly.

   4. The preconceptive dosage of folic acid is _____.

2. Jeannie goes to the pharmacy to buy the folic acid. She also buys several different multivitamins and takes 3 to 4 times the recommended dosage to make sure she will be healthy. What would the nurse tell her about the large dose of vitamins?
   1. "The use of vitamins while pregnant is helpful. Particularly take large doses the first 3 months."
   2. "You only need folic acid; these other pills are just a waste of your money."
   3. "Large doses of vitamins are not recommended and can lead to toxicity."
   4. "You should not be taking any drugs while pregnant."

3. After the baby is born, Jeannie reads about some herbal products that provide contraception and are available in the natural foods store so she doesn't need to visit the midwife or get a prescription. What precautions would the nurse give to Jeannie?
   1. "Herbal products are all dangerous because they are not regulated by the FDA."
   2. "You know these products are OK to take or they wouldn't be advertised on TV."
   3. "You don't need to worry about contraception while you are breastfeeding."
   4. "I would recommend that you consult a midwife or other health care provider for advice about this."

4. Several months after the baby is born, Jeannie develops thrombophlebitis (blood clot in her leg) and is in acute pain. She has read that acupuncture would be a good treatment for this problem. What might the nurse say to Jeannie?
   1. "That is a good idea. What could it hurt to try it?"
   2. "I totally agree. We take too many painkillers as a society."
   3. "What did your doctor recommend?"
   4. "Why don't you experiment and see if you can find something that helps? If not, go to the doctor."

5. Jeannie is diagnosed with thrombophlebitis and started on heparin and then Coumadin. What should the nurse tell her about taking herbal products along with these drugs?
   1. Natural herbal remedies often resolve thrombophlebitis in your legs.
   2. Many herbal products interfere with heparin or Coumadin and might cause bleeding.
   3. You can take herbal products and Coumadin at the same time as long as you eat lots of green vegetables with vitamin K.
   4. There is no problem with drug interactions between natural herbal products and prescription blood thinners.

Preparing and Administering Medications

chapter

7

 Go to http://evolve.elsevier.com/edmunds/lpn/ for additional activities and exercises.

SECTION 1: REVIEW OF MATHEMATICAL PRINCIPLES

See Appendix A for more practice with mathematical principles used in pharmacology.

Nurses who give medications are legally responsible to make sure that the correct dosage is given. There are many health care facilities in which the LPN/LVN works that will require that the nurse calculate the dosage. We know that this seems like a big responsibility, and we want to provide some special mathematical review materials that may be used by those of you who feel that you would benefit from greater study in this area. Some facilities require that a second nurse recheck any math calculation. Be sure that you are aware of the specific policies in your facility as well as in the state in which you practice.

We recommend that you briefly read the review materials and then move through the math calculations. If you find that you are having problems understanding the content or need more practice, there is additional practice at the end of this study guide and on the Evolve website attached to the text. We would also recommend that you use pencil and paper for the calculations, and then repeat the calculations using a calculator.

Some of the tests you will take may require you to manually calculate the math problems.

REVIEW: MULTIPLICATION FACTS

Many students have a need to review basic multiplication and division facts. To assist you in remembering basic math calculations, we have included the table below. Find the two numbers you wish to multiply. Draw a line from the number on the left side of the chart and a line down from the other number in the top column. The answer is where the two lines intersect. Any number times 0 is 0. Any number times 1 is itself.

Multiplication and Division Grid

	2	3	4	5	6	7	8	9	10	11	12
2	4	6	8	10	12	14	16	18	20	22	24
3	6	9	12	15	18	21	24	27	30	33	36
4	8	12	16	20	24	28	32	36	40	44	48
5	10	15	20	25	30	35	40	45	50	55	60
6	12	18	24	30	36	42	48	54	60	66	72
7	14	21	28	35	42	49	56	63	70	77	84
8	16	24	32	40	48	56	64	72	80	88	96
9	18	27	36	45	54	63	72	81	90	99	108
10	20	30	40	50	60	70	80	90	100	110	120
11	22	33	44	55	66	77	88	99	110	121	132
12	24	36	48	60	72	84	96	108	120	132	144

Now calculate the following multiplication problems. Do not use the grid unless you must. Symbols for multiplication include ×, •, or ( ).

1. $9 \times 5 =$

2. $(8)\,(7) =$

3. $7 \bullet 6 =$

4. $(11)\,(4) =$

5. $9 \bullet 3 =$

It is essential to know how to do calculations. Many schools now encourage students to also learn how to use calculators such as small credit card–sized devices, or those on cell phones or computers to do math problems involved in calculating drug dosages. But do not let using a calculator replace using good sense. Always ask yourself if the answer makes sense.

Calculate the math problems in this chapter, and then use calculators to also answer the math problems so you know well how to use both methods to find the correct dosages. If you need help, most calculators come with instructions for doing basic math problems. You may also search online for calculator instructions.

REVIEW: DIVISION FACTS

Divide when you see the symbol ÷ (as $12 \div 4 =$); the symbol — (as $\frac{12}{4}$); the symbol / (as 12/4); or the symbol $\sqrt{}$ (as $4\sqrt{12}$).

Each of these would be read as 12 divided by 4.

In the problem $4\overline{)12}^{\,3}$

The number being divided (12 in the problem above) is called the *dividend*.

The number doing the dividing (4 above) is called the *divisor*.

The number in the answer (3 above) is called the *quotient*.

If the number cannot be divided into equal groups, the number left is the *remainder*. If the remainder is greater than or equal to half the divisor, round the quotient up one number. If it is less than one-half, leave the quotient as it is.

For example:

24	24	24
$25\overline{)600}$	$25\overline{)603}$	$25\overline{)624}$
$\underline{50}$	$\underline{50}$	$\underline{50}$
100	103	124
$\underline{100}$	$\underline{100}$	$\underline{100}$
	$3\ r$	$24\ r$

Therefore, the third quotient will be rounded up to 25.

Look back to the grid reprinted from the text for basic multiplication facts. This grid can also be used for division. On the left side of the chart, find the number you are dividing with. Look across the column for the number you wish to divide. If the number is there, look up the column to find the number that is the exact quotient of the two numbers. If the number is not there, find the closest number. If the number in the chart is slightly larger than the one you want, you will have a remainder. If the number in the chart is slightly smaller, you will have to use a number one less in the quotient. For example, 6 into 42 is exactly 7, while 8 into 50 is 6 with a 2 remainder. Dividing 6 into 29 yields 4 with a 5 remainder.

REVIEW: ROMAN NUMERALS

Roman numerals and their values

I = 1	C = 100
V = 5	D = 500
X = 10	M = 1000
L = 50	

Rules in using Roman numerals

1. Whenever a Roman numeral is repeated, or when a smaller numeral follows a larger one, the values are added together. For example:

    II = 2 (1 + 1 = 2)
    LVII = 57 (50 + 5 +1 + 1 = 57)
    CXIII = 113 (100 + 10 + 1 + 1 + 1 = 113)

2. Whenever a smaller Roman numeral comes before a larger Roman numeral, subtract the smaller value. For example:

    IV = 4 (5 – 1 = 4)
    CD = 400 (500 – 100 = 400)

3. Numerals are never repeated more than three times in a sequence. For example:

    III = 3
    IV = 4

4. Whenever a smaller Roman numeral comes between two larger Roman numerals, subtract the smaller number from the numeral following it. For example:

    XIX = 19 (10 + [10 – 1] = 19)
    XCIX = 99 ([100 – 10] + [10 – 1] = 99)

In expressing dosages in the apothecaries' system, lowercase rather than capital Roman numerals are used. A dot is always placed over the Roman numeral I whenever lowercase numbers are used. For example, iii or vi is the proper form in this system rather than III or VI.

REVIEW: FRACTIONS

A fraction is one or more equal parts of a unit. It is written as two numbers separated by a line, such as 1/2 or 3/4. The parts of the fraction are called the *terms*. The two terms of a fraction are the *numerator* and the *denominator*. The numerator is the top number; the denominator is the bottom number.

$\frac{1}{2}$ = numerator = denominator $\frac{3}{4}$ = numerator = denominator

The denominator tells into how many equal parts the whole has been divided. The numerator tells how many of the parts are being used.

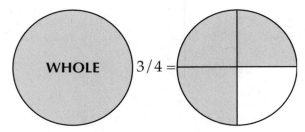

It is important to not confuse these two parts of the fraction. One way to help you remember which part belongs where is to think of the word *nude*. The NUmerator is on top; the DEnominator is on the bottom.

$$\begin{array}{c} N \\ \underline{U} \\ \underline{D} \\ E \end{array}$$

Fractions may be *raised to higher terms* by multiplying both numerator and denominator by the same number. Fractions are *reduced to lower terms* by dividing both terms of the fraction by the same number. The value of the fraction is not changed when it is lowered or raised in terms.

For example:

To raise 3/4 to a higher term, multiply both the numerator and the denominator by 2, converting it to 6/8. The two fractions, 3/4 and 6/8, have the same value.

To lower 3/9 to a lower term, divide both numerator and denominator by 3, converting it to 1/3; 3/9 and 1/3 have the same value.

Proper fractions have a numerator smaller than the denominator. The number 3/4 is a proper fraction because it represents less than 1.

Improper fractions have a numerator the same as or larger than the denominator. The number 6/4 is an improper fraction because the numerator (6) is larger than the denominator (4).

In using fractions in calculations, the numerator and the denominator must be of the same unit of measure. For example, if the numerator is in grains, the denominator must be in grains.

A *mixed number* is a whole number and a proper fraction. Examples of mixed numbers include: 4 1/3; 3 3/4; 5 16/35.

It is often necessary to change an improper fraction to a mixed number or to change a mixed number to an improper fraction when doing certain calculations. To change an improper fraction to a mixed number, divide the denominator into the numerator. The result (quotient) is the whole number. The remainder is placed over the denominator of the improper fraction.

For example: 17/3 is an improper fraction. To convert to a mixed number:

1. Divide the denominator (3) into the numerator (17):

$$
\begin{array}{r}
5 \quad \text{quotient} \\
\text{divisor} \quad 3\,\overline{)\,17} \\
\underline{15} \\
2 \quad \text{remainder}
\end{array}
$$

2. Move the remainder (2) over the denominator (3).

   $\dfrac{2}{3}$ = remainder
   = denominator

3. Put the quotient (5) in front of the fraction.

   5 2/3

To change the mixed number 5 2/3 to an improper fraction, multiply the denominator of the fraction (3) by the whole number (5) add the numerator (2), and place the sum over the denominator. For example:

The sum (17) goes over the denominator of the fraction:

   17/3 is the improper fraction.

A *complex fraction* has a fraction in either its numerator or its denominator, or both. For example:

$$\dfrac{\frac{1}{5}}{50} \quad or \quad \dfrac{30}{\frac{2}{3}} \quad or \quad \dfrac{3\frac{1}{2}}{\frac{1}{8}}$$

Complex fractions may be changed to whole numbers or proper or improper fractions by dividing the number or fraction above the line by the number or fraction below the line.

For example: Change $\dfrac{\frac{1}{2}}{100}$ to a proper fraction as follows:

$$\dfrac{\frac{1}{2}}{100} = \dfrac{1}{2} \div \dfrac{100}{1} = \dfrac{1}{2} \times \dfrac{1}{100} = \dfrac{1}{200}$$

Remember: When dividing fractions, invert or put upside down the divisor and then multiply.

100/1 becomes 1/100.

REVIEW: ADDITION OF FRACTIONS

If fractions have the same denominator, simply add the numerators, and put the sum above the common denominator. For example:

$$\dfrac{2}{12} + \dfrac{3}{12} + \dfrac{5}{12} = \dfrac{10}{12} \quad \dfrac{(sum\ of\ 2+3+5)}{(same\ denominators)}$$

If the fractions have different denominators, they must be converted to a number that each denominator has in common, or a *common denominator*. You can always find a common denominator by multiplying the two denominators by one another. Sometimes, however, both numbers will go into a smaller number. For example: 1/12 + 3/8 + 3/4 = ? What is the smallest common denominator?

1. The smallest whole number that all denominators (12, 8, and 4) have in common is 24; 24, then, is the lowest common denominator.

2. Divide the lowest common denominator by the denominator of each fraction and multiply both terms of the fraction by the quotient (divide 12, 8, and 4 into 24 and multiply the numerator and denominator by the answer). This is often easier to see if we write the problem vertically:

$$\frac{1}{12} = \frac{?}{24} \qquad 24 \div 12 = 2 \qquad \frac{1}{12} \times \frac{2}{2} = \frac{2}{24}$$

$$+\frac{3}{8} = \frac{?}{24} \qquad 24 \div 8 = 3 \qquad \frac{3}{8} \times \frac{3}{3} = \frac{9}{24}$$

$$+\frac{3}{4} = \frac{?}{24} \qquad 24 \div 4 = 6 \qquad \frac{3}{4} \times \frac{6}{6} = \frac{18}{24}$$

3. Then add the numerators and bring down the denominator:

$$\frac{2}{24}$$

$$+\frac{9}{24}$$

$$+\frac{18}{24}$$

$$\frac{29}{24}$$

4. Reduce the improper fraction to its lowest terms by changing the improper fraction to a mixed number.

    $29/24 = 1\ 5/24$

5. If you are adding mixed numbers, first change them to improper fractions and proceed as above.

REVIEW: SUBTRACTION OF FRACTIONS

If fractions have the same denominator, subtract the smaller numerator from the larger numerator. Leave the denominators the same, and then reduce to the lowest terms, if necessary. For example:

$$\frac{5}{10} - \frac{1}{10} = \frac{4}{10} = \frac{2}{5}$$

If fractions do not have the same denominator, change the fractions so they have the smallest common denominator, subtract the numerators, and leave the denominator the same. For example:

$$\frac{15}{28} - \frac{3}{14} = \underline{\qquad}$$

Since 28 is a multiple of 14 ($14 \times 2 = 28$), 28 is a common denominator of 28 and 14. Divide the smallest common denominator by the denominator of each fraction and multiply the numerator and denominator of the fraction by the quotient.

$$\frac{15}{28} = \frac{15}{28} \qquad \text{(no change necessary)}$$

$$- \frac{3}{14} \times \frac{2}{2} = \frac{6}{28}$$

Subtract the numerators and leave the denominators the same.

$$\frac{15}{28} \times \frac{6}{28} = \frac{9}{28}$$

If you are subtracting mixed numbers, first change them to improper fractions and proceed as above.

$2\frac{2}{3} \times 1\frac{1}{28} =$

$\frac{8}{3} \times \frac{7}{6} =$

$\frac{16}{6} \times \frac{7}{6} =$

$\frac{9}{6} \times 1\frac{3}{6} =$

REVIEW: MULTIPLICATION OF FRACTIONS

When multiplying fractions, reduce all to their smallest terms to make calculations simpler. For example, 12/24 is the same as 1/2, but 12/24 is much more difficult to work with. Reducing to the lowest terms is done when you can divide the same number into both the numerator and the denominator (i.e., 2/10 can be divided by 2, therefore 2/10 equals 1/5; 9/36 can be divided by 9, therefore 9/36 equals 1/4).

When the fractions are in their simplest form, multiply the numerators, and then multiply the denominators. For example:

$\frac{1}{20} \times \frac{5}{3} \times 3 =$

Remember . . .

Because 3 is a whole number it is the same as 3/1.
The 1 can be added as a denominator if it makes it easier to understand.

By reducing any numerator with any denominator, this can be simplified as follows:

$$\frac{1}{20} \times \frac{5}{3} \times 3 = \frac{1}{4} \times \frac{1}{3} \times \frac{3}{1}$$
$$= \frac{3}{12}$$
$$= \frac{1}{4}$$

If the number is a mixed number (a whole number and a fraction), change it to an improper fraction before solving. For example:

$$2\frac{1}{2} \times \frac{2}{3} \times 6 = \frac{5}{2} \times \frac{2}{3} \times \frac{6}{1}$$
Simplify: $= \frac{5}{1} \times \frac{1}{1} \times \frac{2}{1}$
$$= \frac{10}{1}$$
$$= 10$$

REVIEW: DIVISION OF FRACTIONS

To divide a fraction by a fraction, invert (or turn upside down) the divisor and then multiply and reduce answers to lowest terms.

For example:

$$\frac{4}{6} \quad \div \quad \frac{2}{6} \quad = \quad ?$$

Invert the divisor.

$$\frac{\cancel{4}^2}{\cancel{6}_1} \quad \times \quad \frac{\cancel{6}^1}{\cancel{2}_1} \quad = \quad ?$$

Simplify, then multiply numerators and then denominators.

$$\frac{4}{6} \quad \times \quad \frac{6}{2} \quad = \quad ?$$

$$\frac{2}{1} \quad \times \quad \frac{1}{1} \quad = \quad \frac{2}{1} \quad = \quad 2$$

If the number is a mixed number, change it to an improper fraction before solving. For example:

$$\frac{2}{3} \quad \div \quad 1\frac{1}{3} \quad = \quad ?$$

Change mixed number to an improper fraction:

$$\frac{2}{3} \quad \div \quad \frac{4}{3} \quad = \quad ?$$

Invert divisor:

$$\frac{\cancel{2}^1}{\cancel{3}_1} \quad \times \quad \frac{\cancel{3}^1}{\cancel{4}_2} \quad = \quad ?$$

Simplify:

$$\frac{2}{3} \quad \times \quad \frac{3}{4} \quad = \quad ?$$

$$\frac{1}{1} \quad \times \quad \frac{1}{2} \quad = \quad \frac{1}{2}$$

REVIEW: DECIMAL FRACTIONS

A decimal fraction is one whose denominator is 10 or some multiple of 10. Instead of writing the denominator, a decimal point is added to the numerator.

For example:

$$1/4 = 25/100 = 0.25$$

All numbers to the left of the decimal point represent whole numbers. Those numbers to the right represent fractions. Zeros may be placed to the right of the decimal for a whole number only, without changing the value of the whole number (i.e., 45 is the same as 45.0 or 45.00).

Decimals increase in value from right to left; they decrease in value from left to right. Decimals increase in value in multiples of 10. Each column in a decimal has its own value, according to where it lies from the decimal point (see the figure below).

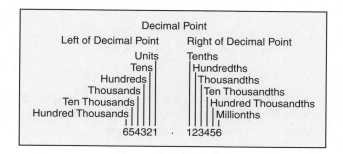

Addition and Subtraction of Decimal Fractions:

Place the numbers so that the decimal points fall in a straight line. Keep the columns straight. Add zeros to the right after the decimal point, if necessary. Then add or subtract as you would for whole numbers. The decimal point goes in the answer just below the decimal points in the problem.

For example: add 0.0678 and 1.082

```
   0.0678
+  1.0820   (add one zero)
   1.1498
```

The decimal point is in line with the other decimal points. Subtract 3.053 from 6.046:

```
   6.046
-  3.053
   2.993
```

Multiplication and Division of Decimal Fractions:

To multiply decimal fractions, multiply the two numbers and count off from right to left as many decimal places in the product (answer) as there were in the multiplier and multiplicand. For example:

```
   44.61        Multiplicand (has 2 decimal places)
  × 2.3         Multiplier (has 1 decimal place)
  13383
   8922
 102.603        Count off 3 places right to left and insert a decimal point. If you do not have enough places,
                add zeros in front of the numbers.
```

To divide by a decimal fraction, first move the decimal point in the divisor (the number you are dividing with) enough places right to make it a whole number. Then move the decimal point in the dividend (the number you are dividing) as many places as it was moved in the divisor, adding zeros if necessary. Place the decimal point in the quotient (answer) directly above that in the dividend.

For example: divide 32.80 by 8.2.

$8.2\overline{)32.80}$ 8.2 is the divisor; 32.80 is the dividend

Move the decimal point in the divisor to the right to make it a whole number, then move it the same number of places in the dividend.

$82.\overline{)328.0}$

Solve the problem:

$$82.\overline{)328.0}\quad\begin{array}{r}4.0\\\hline\end{array}$$
$$328.0$$

Because the decimal system is built on multiples of 10, a shortcut may be taken when multiplying or dividing by 10, 100, or 1000. To multiply a decimal fraction by 10, 100, or 1000, move the decimal place as many places to the right as there are zeros in the multiplier. For example:

$$0.0006 \times 1000 = ?$$
In 1000 there are three zeros, so
$$0.0006 \times 1000 = 0000.6 = 0.6$$

To divide a decimal fraction by 10, 100, or 1000, move the decimal place as many places to the left as there are zeros in the divisor. For example:

$$0.5/100 = ?$$
100 has 2 whole number zeros, so
$$0.5/100 = 0.005$$

REVIEW: RATIOS AND PERCENTS

Ratios

A *ratio* is a way of expressing the relationship of one number to another number or of expressing a part of a whole number. The relationship is expressed by separating the numbers with a colon (:). The colon means division. The expression 1:2 is read as there is one part to two parts. Ratios are commonly used to express concentrations of a drug in solution.

For example, a ratio written as 1:20 means 1 part to 20 parts. A ratio may also be written as a fraction (e.g., 1:10 is the same as 1/10).

Percent

The term *percent* or the symbol % means parts per hundred. Thus, the percentage may also be expressed as a fraction or as a decimal fraction. For example:

30% means 30 parts per hundred or 30/100
70% means 70 parts per hundred or 70/100

Percents should also be reduced to their lowest common denominator, when appropriate. For example:

20% is 20/100 or 1/5
40% is 40/100 or 2/5

To *change a fraction to a percent*, divide the numerator by the denominator and multiply the results (quotient) by 100 and add a percent sign (%). For example:

To change 8/10 to a percent:
$8 \div 10 = 0.8$
$0.8 \times 100 = 80\%$

To change 2/5 to a percent:
$2 \div 5 = 0.4$
$0.4 \times 100 = 40\%$

To *change a mixed number to a percent*, first change it to an improper fraction, then proceed as above. For example:

To change 1 1/3 to a percent:

$$4/3 = 4 \div 3 = 1.33 \text{ remainder } 1$$
$$1.33 \times 100 = 133\ 1/3\%$$

To *change a ratio to a percent*, the ratio is first expressed as a fraction. The first number or term of the ratio becomes the numerator and the second number or term becomes the denominator (e.g., 1:200 becomes 1/200). The fraction is then changed to a percent as shown above.

$$1:200 = 1/200$$
$$1 \div 200 = 0.005$$
$$0.005 \times 100 = 0.5\%$$

To *change a percent to a ratio*, the percent becomes the numerator and is placed over the denominator of 100.

For example, to change 20% and 50% to ratios:

$$20\% \text{ is } 20/100 = 1/5 \text{ or } 1:5$$
$$50\% \text{ is } 50/100 = 1/2 \text{ or } 1:2$$

A percent may easily be expressed as a decimal, a fraction or as a ratio.

Example: $20\% = 0.20 = 20/100 = 1/5 = 1:5$

It is very easy to change between decimals, fractions, percents, and ratios. The following rules are presented to summarize these changes:

Rules for Changing Between Percents, Decimals, Fractions, and Ratios

To *change a fraction to a ratio*, write the two numbers with a colon between them instead of the dividing line.

Example: $1/5 = 1:5$

To *change a fraction to a decimal fraction*, divide the numerator by the denominator.

Example: $1/5 = 0.20$

To *change a fraction to a percent*, divide the numerator by the denominator (use as many decimal places as needed); then move the decimal point two places to the right and add the percent sign.

Example: $1/5 = 0.20 = 20\%$

To *change a percent to a decimal fraction*, move the decimal point two places to the left and omit the percent sign.

Example: $10\% = 0.10$

To *change a percent to a fraction*, drop the percent sign, write the number as the numerator, with 100 as the denominator, and reduce to the lowest terms.

Example: $10\% = 10/100 = 1/10$

To *change a percent to a ratio*, drop the percent sign, use the number as the first term, 100 as the second term, and reduce to the lowest terms; or change to a fraction and then use a colon instead of the dividing line.

Example: $10\% = 10/100 = 1/10$ or 1:10
$10\% = 1/10 = 1:10$

To *change a decimal fraction to a percent*, move the decimal point two places to the right (multiply by 100) and add the percent sign.

Example: $0.20 = 20\%$

To *change a decimal fraction to a common fraction*, omit the decimal point and place the number over the appropriate denominator of 10, 100, or 1000, and reduce to the lowest terms.

Example: $0.20 = 20/100 = 1/5$

To *change a decimal fraction to a ratio*, write the number as the first term; then put 10, 100, or 1000 as the second term; finally, reduce to the lowest terms.

Example: $0.20 = 20{:}100$ or 1:5

To *change a ratio to a fraction*, write the numbers with a dividing line instead of a colon.

Example: $1{:}20 = 1/20$

To *change a ratio to a decimal fraction*, divide the first term by the second term.

Example: $1{:}20 = 0.05$

To *change a ratio to a percent*, divide the first term by the second term, move the decimal point two places to the right in the answer, and add a percent sign.

Example: $1{:}20 = 0.05 = 5\%$

REVIEW: PROPORTIONS

A proportion is a way of expressing a relationship of equality between two ratios. In other words, the first ratio listed is equal to the second ratio listed. The two ratios are separated by a double colon (::), which means, "as." The numbers of each end of the relationship are the extremes, and the two numbers in the middle are the means. *The product of the extremes equals the product of the means.* This means that if one of the terms is not known, it may be calculated. The unknown term is defined by an x. For example:

$$5 : 500 :: 2 : x$$

(when x is the unknown) means

"The relationship of 5 to 500 is the same as the relationship of 2 to x."

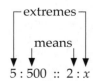

5 and x are the extremes; 500 and 2 are the means.

Proportions may be written as fractions. To find x, express the proportion as a relationship, and solve:

$$5/500 = 2/x$$
$$2 \times 500 = 1000$$
$$5x = 1000$$
$$x = 1000/5$$
$$x = 200$$

In addition to being equal, proportions must also be written in the same system in both ratios (e.g., minims is to grains as minims is to grains; mL is to grams as mL is to grams). For example:

$$15 \text{ m} : 60 \text{ gr} :: 13 \text{ m} : x \text{ gr} \quad \text{Correctly written}$$
$$15 \text{ m} : 60 \text{ m} :: 13 \text{ m} : x \text{ gr} \quad \text{Incorrectly written}$$

The calculation of ratios provides one of the major foundations in drug dosage calculation. Often the nurse knows the desired concentration of a drug and needs to calculate how much to give of a medication on hand. The nurse can figure how much medication to give by using the principles of proportion.

SECTION 2: MATHEMATICAL EQUIVALENTS USED IN PHARMACOLOGY

See Appendix B for more practice with mathematical equivalents used in pharmacology.

REVIEW: COMMON MEASURES

Common Household Equivalents

1 teaspoon = approximately 5 mL
1 tablespoon = 3 teaspoons
1 cup = 8 ounces
1 pint = 2 cups
1 quart = 4 cups

Other Common Measures

Other common measures include inch, foot, and yard, as well as ounce or pound.

2.2 lb = 1 kg or 1000 g
1 inch = 25.4 millimeters
1 foot = 0.3 meters
1 yard = 1.61 kilometers
1 ounce = 28.35 grams
1 pound = 0.45 kilogram

The Apothecaries' System

The apothecaries' system is no longer in great use. A few components remain for some products:

1 grain = 60 or 64 mg or 0.06 g; 1/60 grain = 1 mg

To convert grains to grams, divide by 15 or 16. To convert grams to milligrams, move the decimal point three places to the right. To convert grams to grains, multiply by 15 or 16.

To convert grains to milligrams, multiply by 60 or 64. To convert milligrams to grams, move the decimal point three places to the left. To convert milligrams to grains, divide by 60 or 64.

Common Measurements in the Metric System

Measures of Length (Meter)
1 meter (m) = 100 centimeters (cm)
1 centimeter (cm) = 0.01 meter (m)

Measures of Volume (Liter)
1 decaliter (d) = 10 liters (L)
1 liter (L) = 1000 milliliters (mL) or 1000 cubic centimeters (cc)

Measures of Weight (Gram)
1 kilogram (kg) = 1000 grams (g)
1 gram (g) = 1000 milligrams (mg)
1 milligram (mg) = 1000 micrograms (µg or mcg)

Key Point: Cubic centimeters, milliliters, and grams are approximately equivalent; 1 cc or 1 mL weighs approximately 1 g.

1 cc = 1 mL = 1 g, whereas 1 kg = 2.2 lbs

Relying on what you know about the decimal system, you can change measures within the same system:

To change milligrams to micrograms:

Move decimal point three places to right. 000.00007 mg = 000000.07 mcg

To change micrograms to milligrams:

Move decimal point three places to left. 000000.07 mcg = 000.00007 mg

To change grams to milligrams:

Move decimal point three places to the right (multiply by 1000). 1.000067 g = 1000.067 mg

To change milligrams to grams:

Move decimal point three places to the left (divide by 1000). 1345.0789 mg = 1.3450789 g

Key Point: Prefixes of the metric system indicate the multiples or fractions of the unit:

milli = one-thousandth
deca = ten
centi = one-hundredth
hecto = hundred
deci = one-tenth
kilo = thousand

REVIEW: COMMON MEASURES

Equivalents in the Apothecaries' and Metric Systems*

Apothecaries' System		Metric System
1 gallon (gal)	=	4000 cc or 4000 mL or 4 L
1 qt or 32 oz	=	1000 cc or 1000 mL or 1 L
1 pt or 16 oz	=	500 cc or 500 mL or 500 g
15-16 grains, or 15-16 minims	=	1 cc or 1 mL or 1 g
2.2 lbs	=	1000 g or 1 kg
1 grain	=	60 or 64 mg or 0.06 g
1/60 grain	=	1 mg

*To aid in teaching the conversion processes, some approximations have been made in these equivalencies. In addition, 15 rather than 16 grains are often used in calculations; 60 is often used in place of 64. These approximations account for the variance seen in the table.

Rules for Converting from One System to Another

Units to Change	Method
Grains to grams	Divide by 15 or 16.
Grains to milligrams	Multiply by 60 or 64.
Grams to grains	Multiply by 15 or 16.
Grams to milligrams	Move decimal point three places to the right.
Milligrams to grains	Divide by 60 or 64.
Milligrams to grams	Move decimal point three places to left.
Minims to cubic centimeters	Divide by 15 or 16.

REVIEW: CONVERTING TEMPERATURE READINGS BETWEEN CENTIGRADE (CELSIUS) AND FAHRENHEIT SCALES

The key relationships to understand are:
- One degree on the Fahrenheit scale equals 9/5 of one degree on the Celsius scale.
- One degree on the Celsius scale equals 5/9 of one degree on the Fahrenheit scale.

The formula for converting Fahrenheit to Celsius is: $(°F - 32) \times 5/9 = °C$

For example,

Change 98° F to degrees Celsius (round to the nearest tenth degree):

$(°F - 32) \times 5/9 = °C$
$(98° - 32) = 66 \times 5/9 = 36.7° C$

The formula for converting Celsius to Fahrenheit is: $(°C \times 9/5) + 32 = °F$

For example,

Change 38.8° C to degrees Fahrenheit (round to the nearest tenth degree):

$(°C \times 9/5) + 32 = °F$
$(38.8° \times 9/5) + 32 = 101.8° C$

SECTION 3: CALCULATING DRUG DOSAGES

See Appendix C for more practice calculating drug dosages.

REVIEW: COMPUTING ORAL DOSAGES THROUGH RATIO-PROPORTION

The formula to calculate the number of capsules or tablets to order is a basic proportion problem (review proportions in textbook, Chapter 7):

$$\frac{\text{Dose ordered}}{\text{Dose available}} \quad :: \quad \frac{\text{Tablets or capsules per dose}}{\text{Drug form (tablets or capsules)}} \quad = \quad \text{Number of tablets or capsules per dose}$$

Key Point:

1. First change dosages to the same unit of measurement.
2. Reduce to simplest terms.
3. Use common sense to check your answer.

Remember: When parentheses are used in a math problem, it means to do all the calculations inside the parentheses first, then complete the rest of the problem.

The formula is the same for calculating liquid dosages. Only the unit of measure is different. For liquids, use:

$$\frac{\text{Dose desired}}{\text{Dose available}} \quad \times \quad \text{Drug form (minims, mL, dram)} \quad = \quad \text{Amount of liquid per dose}$$

REVIEW: COMPUTING DOSAGES OF PARENTERAL MEDICATIONS

Ratio and proportion are the standard methods of calculating parenteral dosages.

Drug available : Dilution :: Drug desired : x

$$\frac{\text{Dose desired}}{\text{Dose available}} \quad \times \quad \text{Dilution or amount of solution} \quad = \quad \text{Amount of solution per dose}$$

If instructions are not given for diluting medications, a modification of the familiar proportion formula may be used:

$$\text{Dose desired} : 1 \text{ mL} :: \text{Total drug available} : x$$

Note: This is not the Desired/Available formula we have been using. Desired does not always go over Available. Think about what you are looking for!

Look at the relationships in the formula:

$$\text{Dose desired} : 1 \text{ mL} :: \text{Total drug available} : x$$

Dose to known amount of liquid compared to dose to unknown amount of liquid.

Multiply the means, divide by the extremes.

$$\frac{\text{Total drug available}}{\text{Dose desired}} \quad \times \quad 1 \text{ mL} \quad = \quad \begin{array}{l}\text{Amount of diluent required}\\\text{to add vial powder so that}\\\text{dose ordered} = 1 \text{ mL}\end{array}$$

Another time when solutions are involved is when sterile hypodermic tablets are to be administered. These special tablets are placed in a syringe and diluted, usually with 1 mL solution. The amount to be given may be computed thus:

Amount available : 1 mL :: Amount desired : x mL

REVIEW: COMPUTING DOSAGES OF INSULIN

The calculation and preparation of insulin dosage is unique in three ways:

1. There are many different kinds of insulin, but they all come in a standardized measure called a *unit*. Insulin is available in 10 mL vials in two strengths: U-100 (100 units per 1 mL solution) or U-500 (500 units per 1 mL solution). U-500 is five times stronger than U-100. (U-500 is rarely used.)

2. Insulin should be drawn up in a special insulin syringe calibrated in units.

   For example, the order reads *"80 units of regular (Iletin) U-100 insulin."* When this insulin is to be given in a TB syringe, the dosage calculation is:

   $$\frac{\text{Dose desired}}{\text{Dose available}} = \frac{80 \text{ units}}{100 \text{ units}} \times 16 \text{ minims} = \frac{64}{5} = 12.8 \text{ minims}$$

3. The insulin order, the insulin bottle, and the insulin as drawn up should always be rechecked by another nurse for maximum accuracy. Small errors may cause big problems!

REVIEW: CALCULATING FLOW RATES FOR INTRAVENOUS INFUSIONS

Many hospitals or other health care facilities will use special machines to calculate the flow rate for IV fluids. However, many nursing homes or other settings may not have this type of expensive equipment and so the LPN/LVN may need to be able to calculate these problems.

1. Calculating the flow rate for IV fluid administration.
   A. The rate at which IV fluids are given is the *flow rate* and is measured in drops per minute.
   B. *Drop factor* is the number of drops per milliliter of liquid and is determined by the size of the drops.

The drop factor is different for different manufacturers of IV infusion equipment and must be checked by reading it on the infusion set label. Generally, though, drop factors range between 10 and 15 drops per milliliter. Infusion sets have different drop factors for use with blood infusion sets (usually 10 to 12 drops per milliliter) because the drops are larger, while pediatric setups use very small drops called *microdrops* (often with 50 or 60 microdrops per milliliter).

Key Point: The flow rate for infusions can be calculated.

The drop factor for infusions depends upon the type of equipment and must be read from the infusion set label.

Once the nurse has learned the drop factor for the equipment being used, the flow rate may be calculated by using the following formula:

Drop factor × Milliliters per minute = Flow rate (drops/min)

or

$$\frac{\text{Total of fluid to give}}{\text{Total time (minutes)}} \times \text{Drop factor} = \text{Flow rate (drops/min)}$$

2. Modifying the drop rate for children.

The drop factor must be determined from the infusion setup. Usually 60 microdrops per mL is the drop factor for infants. For calculating the flow rates in infants, the same formula is used, except the microdrop drop factor must be substituted into the formula for the adult drop factor.

$$\frac{\text{Total of fluid to give}}{\text{Total time (minutes)}} \times \text{Drop factor} = \text{Flow rate (drops/min)}$$

3. Calculating total administration time.

Sometimes physicians will specify how fast they want infusions to run. The nurse needs to calculate the total time the infusion will run.

Calculating total administration time for IV fluid depends on calculating the total number of drops to be infused. Using this information, plus the drop factor, the total infusion time can easily be determined by use of the following formula:

$$\frac{\text{Total drops to be infused}}{\text{Flow rate (drops/min)} \times 60} = \text{Total infusion time (hr or min)}$$

REVIEW: COMPUTING DOSAGES FOR INFANTS AND CHILDREN

1. *Clark's rule*: Based on the child's body weight.

   Based on the proportion of the average adult weight and the adult dosage, we can calculate the child's dosage using the child's weight.

   Adult weight : Adult dosage :: Child's weight : *x* (Child's dosage)

   $$\frac{\text{Weight of the child}}{\text{Weight of the adult}} \times \text{Adult dose} = \text{Child's dose}$$

Some instructors may substitute kilograms for pounds in calculating the weight, but the formula remains the same. To convert pounds into kilograms, divide the weight of the adult and the weight of the child by 2.2 to obtain weight in kilograms.

2. *Body surface area*: Used for children when accuracy is needed. The total body surface area is determined using a nomogram or chart (see following page), and is put into the following formula:

$$\frac{\text{Surface area of the child in square meters}}{\text{Surface area of an adult in square meters (1.73 m}^2)} \times \text{Usual adult dose} = \text{Child's dose}$$

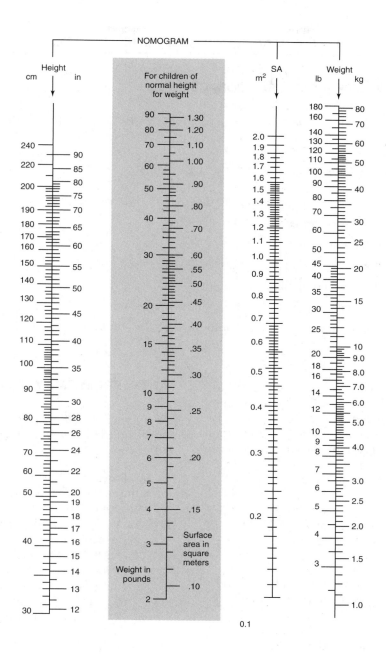

NOMOGRAM

BSA nomogram. Place a straight edge from the patient's height in the left column to his or her weight in the right column. The point of intersection on the body surface area column indicates the body surface area (BSA).

(From Lilley LL, Harrington S, Snyder JS: *Pharmacology and the Nursing Process*, ed 5, St Louis, 2007, Mosby; modified from data by Boyd E, West CD, in Berhman RE, Kliegman RM, Jensen HB: *Nelson textbook of pediatrics*, ed 17, Philadelphia, 2004, W.B. Saunders.)

SECTION 4: PREPARING AND ADMINISTERING MEDICATIONS

PART I: RECOGNIZING DIFFERENT ORAL DOSAGE FORMS

Major concept to understand: There is always a particular reason why a medication is given by a route other than the oral route.

Match the following words with the proper descriptions.

1. _____ A liquid with a high sugar content to disguise the bitter taste
2. _____ A dried powder compressed into small pellets
3. _____ A medication that is sucked
4. _____ A liquid that you shake prior to pouring
5. _____ A medication with high alcohol content
6. _____ Gelatin containers that must not be opened or crushed
7. _____ A medication that contains an agent to increase the solubility

   a. capsules
   b. elixirs
   c. suspensions
   d. lozenges
   e. tablets
   f. emulsions
   g. syrups

8. A patient was asking her nurse why she had to take her medications by mouth. What are possible things the nurse might say?
   1. "Medications that are ordered by your doctor are usually given by mouth and easier to take."
   2. "Medications taken by mouth are always the least expensive.
   3. "All medications are given by mouth unless they need to be given stat IV."
   4. "A generic medication must always be taken by mouth."

9. Important considerations to remember when giving oral medications include steps that must be taken. Place in the correct order the following steps in administering oral medications.
   1. Compare the dosage ordered to the label on the container.
   2. Clarify the drug order if confusing.
   3. Do not touch the medication with your hands.
   4. Explain to your patient what you are giving and answer questions.
   5. Document the medications that you have given.
   6. Check the identity of your patient.

   _____, _____, _____, _____, _____, _____

PART II: PROBLEMS WITH IV INFUSIONS

Major concept to understand: Develop a checklist in your head to follow when trying to figure out why an IV is not running well.

1. Ms. Jones calls the nurse because her IV is not running well. She has just returned from the bathroom, and the IV bag is lying on the bed. What actions will the nurse need to take to correct the problem?
   1. Observe the arm to see what the IV site looks like.
   2. Hang the IV bag back up on the pole and the problem should be solved.
   3. Leave the bag where it is and call the RN to check it.
   4. Discontinue the IV.

2. Mr. Harry mentions that after his bed bath, his arm began burning where the IV is inserted. What actions will the nurse need to take to correct the problem?
   1. Observe the arm to see what the IV site looks like.
   2. Speed up the IV to stop it from burning.
   3. Increase the IV rate to flush out the air.
   4. Discontinue the IV.

3. Terry Brown, age 3, has begun to cry, pulling at the IV in his arm. The IV infusion site is reddened. What is the most likely problem causing the pain?
   1. air embolism
   2. disconnected IV
   3. infiltration of IV site
   4. kinked tubing

4. The alarm on the IV infusion pump for Mr. King begins to sound. The nurse enters the room and finds air in the tubing. What will the nurse do next?
   1. Discontinue the IV.
   2. Call the physician.
   3. Increase the IV rate to flush out the air.
   4. Stop the IV, remove air from line, restart the IV.

5. Ms. Wallace is a very obese patient with a broken hip. She is unable to get out of bed. The nurse notices that her IV is not dripping. What would the nurse check to correct the problem?
   1. Check the IV site.
   2. See if she needs new IV tubing.
   3. Check the rate of the IV infusion.
   4. Check the patient's temperature.

PART III: WORKING WITH PARENTERAL AND PERCUTANEOUS PRODUCTS

1. What are some reasons for nurses to give medications by the parenteral route? (Select all that apply.)
   1. The patient refuses to take oral medications.
   2. The medication must be given as a patch.
   3. The medication is not compatible with stomach acid.
   4. The patient is unable to take oral medications.

2. What are the most common sites for intramuscular injections? (Select all that apply.)
   1. deltoid
   2. vastus lateralis
   3. triceps
   4. gastrocnemius
   5. dorsogluteal
   6. quadriceps

3. The physician has ordered an antibiotic to be given to a very ill patient hospitalized with pneumonia. What route would the nurse expect the order to specify?
   1. as an ointment
   2. in the form of a nebulizer
   3. as an IV piggyback
   4. as an oral medication

4. Needle gauge measurements are related to what part of the needle?
   1. shaft
   2. internal diameter
   3. length
   4. beveled tip

5. Parenteral medications come in the following forms: (Select all that apply.)
   1. closed-loop systems
   2. suppositories
   3. ampules
   4. Mix-O-Vials

PART IV: USING STANDARD PRECAUTIONS IN GIVING MEDICATIONS

Major concept to understand: Not only must the nurse act to protect the patient when he or she is giving medications, but also must act to protect him- or herself.

Mr. Green was brought to the emergency department by the emergency medical technicians (EMTs). He was found in an alley and was drunk and confused and has a large lump on his head. While the nurse is washing his skin with alcohol to start an IV, Mr. Green becomes incontinent of feces, which gets all over the nurse's clothing and arms.

1. How would the nurse evaluate the risk of exposure to HIV or hepatitis B virus?
   1. Very high because your skin came into direct contact with feces
   2. Low for HIV, but very high for hepatitis B virus
   3. Very low because HIV and hepatitis B virus are blood-borne pathogens
   4. Low because the exposure to feces was not very extensive

2. Mr. Green begins to vomit. The vomitus is clear with streaks of bright-red blood. Does this change the evaluation of risk?
   1. No, the gastric juices inactivate the HIV and hepatitis B virus.
   2. No, vomitus is not an implicated fluid for HIV or hepatitis B.
   3. No, vomitus is not potentially infectious in this situation.
   4. Yes, the contamination of vomitus with blood increases the risk of HIV or hepatitis B infection.

3. The nurse just gave Mr. Green an antibiotic by injection. What special precautions should be taken?
   1. Recap the needle and dispose of it in a puncture-resistant container located in the patient's room.
   2. Use gloves when giving the injection. Dispose of the needle in a puncture-resistant container located in the patient's room.
   3. Make certain to bend the needle so that it cannot be used again.
   4. Use the triceps muscle, then wash your hands with soap and water after giving the injection.

4. Mr. Green has had numerous past admissions. When the old chart arrives, the nurse finds that he does have a positive test for HIV. How will this affect the nurse's care for this patient?
   1. The nurse should wear gloves and protective barriers when performing procedures that may produce blood, take precautions to prevent injuries from needles, and wash hands and surfaces immediately with soap and warm water if they are contaminated with blood or other body fluids.
   2. The nurse refuses to care for him because she does not want any further exposure to HIV.
   3. The nurse should wear gloves, mask, and gown whenever she enters the room. She should also make sure visitors do the same.
   4. The nurse does not need to take any special precautions with him, except to wear a gown.

5. In giving Mr. Green his next dose of antibiotic, the nurse accidentally sticks herself with the needle. The nurse should:
   1. immediately scrub the area vigorously with a strong disinfectant soap and leave for the day.
   2. wash the area and fill out an incident report for the nursing supervisor.
   3. wash the area and follow the institution's procedure for reporting the incident and follow-up treatment.
   4. wash the area. The nurse was giving an antibiotic so the risk of any infection to her is very small. The institutional policy makes it optional whether she reports it or not.

PART V: ETHICAL-LEGAL SITUATIONS TO PONDER IN PREPARING AND ADMINISTERING MEDICATIONS

1. Nurse Fairland has been preparing some Demerol for Mr. Jones, a patient who is in pain. Another of her patients is just returning from surgery and needs to be put to bed. Nurse Fairland asks you to give Mr. Jones the pain medication she has just drawn up while she helps the patient returning from surgery. How will you respond to the request?
   1. "I have other things to do. He's your patient, you do it."
   2. "I would love to help you, so why don't I help your surgical patient instead?"
   3. "Sure, no problem."
   4. "I think you need to take care of your own patients. I have enough of my own."

2. Why did you choose that answer?

3. The nurse has worked on this medical unit for weeks and knows all of the patients well. When she begins to give medications, she notices that Mr. Glenn isn't wearing an identification bracelet. He is older and confused, but she knows him well. What will be the nurse's next action?
   1. Give him his medications, then get a new identification bracelet.
   2. Refuse to give him his medications until he finds his bracelet.
   3. Give him his mediations because he is responding to you.
   4. Get him a new identification bracelet then give him his medications.

4. Why did you choose that answer?

5. The nurse arrives in Mrs. Babcock's room just as her husband comes to visit. Mrs. Babcock wants to walk in the hallway and asks the nurse to leave her Lanoxin on the bedside table. "I'll take it when I get back." she says. What will the nurse say?
   1. "Okay, I will leave it here for you to take when you get back."
   2. "I think it best if I keep it with me until you get back."
   3. "I insist you take this before you go for your walk."
   4. "I will take it to the medication room and bring it to you when you get back."

6. Why did you choose that answer?

7. The nurse accidentally stuck himself with a needle after giving a patient an injection. No one saw this happen. What should the nurse do now?
   1. Report the needlestick and follow agency policies regarding incident reporting.
   2. Keep the accident to himself; it really will not affect him.
   3. Ask the patient if he or she has any diseases like hepatitis or AIDS.
   4. Wash his hands and ask the patient to wash his or her hands also.

8. Why did you choose that answer?

REVIEW: READING DRUG LABELS

Drug labels are required on all medication containers. The label must indicate the contents and the directions for its administration. When medications are packaged in the unit dose system, only one dose is provided in each package. The medication is not removed from the packaging until the medication is given to the patient.

By law, the drug label is required to list the following types of information:
- Drug name
- Dosage strength
- Formulation of medication: tablet, capsule, etc.
- Total amount per bottle or vial
- Manufacturer
- Instructions for storage or reconstitution
- Expiration date

Look at the following label:

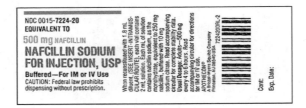

When only one name is listed—for example, nafcillin sodium—this indicates a generic name. If there were a trade name listed on *this* label, nafcillin sodium would be listed in a smaller type underneath the trade name.

The drug label says "for injection" and further states that it is for IV or IM use. This makes it clear that it cannot be given orally.

The drug label also states that this is 500 mg nafcillin. The small type indicates the dosage per mL when the product is reconstituted and lists the usual adult dosage.

PART VI: PRACTICE READING DRUG LABELS

Look at the following label and determine:

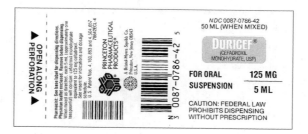

1. What are the generic and trade names of the medication?

2. How is this product to be administered?

3. What is the total mL in the bottle when mixed?

4. What is the dosage/mL when mixed?

5. Who is the manufacturer?

Look at the next label:

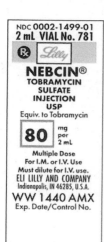

6. What are the generic and trade names of the medication?

7. How is this product to be administered?

8. What is the total mL in the bottle when mixed?

9. What is the dosage per mL?

10. Who is the manufacturer?

Look at the next label:

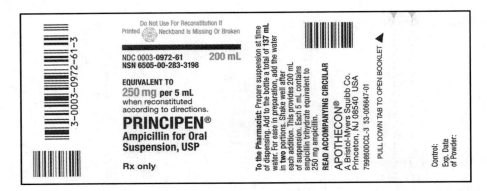

11. What are the generic and trade names of the medication?

12. How is this product to be administered?

13. What is the total mL in the bottle?

14. What is the dosage per mL?

15. How many mL contain 500 mg?

16. What is the total mg in the bottle?

PART VII: MASTERING IMPORTANT CONCEPTS IN PREPARING AND ADMINISTERING MEDICATIONS

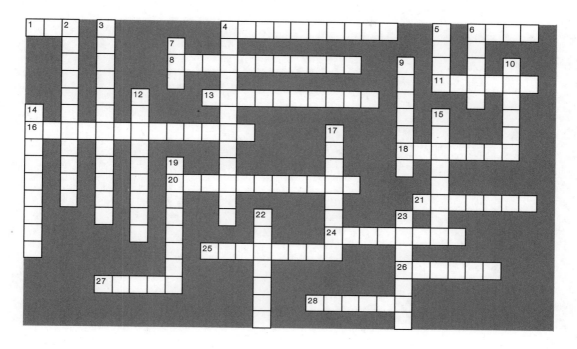

Across

1. The portion of a syringe that holds the needle.
4. The _____ route is into the skin, can be intradermal, Sub Q or IM.
6. Term often used by patients to describe a capsule or tablet.
8. This route is used when it is necessary for the medication to enter the bloodstream directly.
11. Applied against the inside of the cheek.
13. Applied under the tongue.
16. The medication is deposited deep into the muscle mass.
18. _____ medications are applied directly to the area of skin requiring treatment.
20. A _____ (NG) tube is another route for enteral medication.
21. Liquids made up of drugs dissolved in alcohol and water.
24. Particles of medication or pieces of a blood clot that break loose and travel in the patient's bloodstream.
25. Medicine mixed with a hard sugar base and are sucked on.
26. Portion of the syringe that includes the hub, shaft and tip which pierces the skin.
27. Single or multiple-dose glass containers of medication.
28. Contains one dose of medication in a small, breakable glass container.

Down

2. Always follow infection control _____.
3. Placing < 2 mL of fluid into the loose tissue between the dermis and muscle layer.
4. Topical application of medication for absorption through the skin.
5. Injecting a small volume creates a bump like a mosquito bite and is called a _____.
6. A nitroglycerine _____ adheres to the skin with adhesive edges.
7. A two-compartment vial is called a _____-o-vial.
9. Dried, powdered drugs compressed into small shapes.
10. The portion of a syringe that contains the medication.
12. Solutions that have small droplets of water and medication dispersed in oil.
14. A second IV container that is hung slightly higher than the first IV.
15. Gelatin containers that hold powder or liquid medicine.
17. Instruments for injecting liquids.
19. Metered-dose _____ deliver medication to nasal or lung tissue.
22. Prevention of infection.
23. The inner portion of a syringe that fits into the barrel.

Allergy and Respiratory Medications

chapter

8

 Go to http://evolve.elsevier.com/edmunds/lpn/ for additional activities and exercises.

PART I: ANTIHISTAMINES

1. Histamine, a chemical produced by the body:
   1. is released in response to mast cells and basophils.
   2. is released only when infection is present.
   3. produces the inflammatory response in the body.
   4. acts to relieve the erythema and swelling caused by inflammation.

2. Antihistamines act to competitively block the action of:
   1. histamine by producing vasodilation and increased capillary permeability.
   2. histamine by competing with it for receptor sites.
   3. acetylcholine by occupying the H_1 receptor sites at effector structures.
   4. anticholinergic receptors in effector structures.

3. *Seasonal allergic rhinitis* refers to:
   1. colds that develop only during the winter.
   2. a runny nose in the summer.
   3. a runny nose caused by perennial allergic phenomena.
   4. an allergy that develops during holidays when surrounded by many people.

4. The adverse reaction most commonly associated with antihistamines is:
   1. tachycardia.
   2. difficult urination.
   3. insomnia.
   4. sedation.

5. The use of central nervous system (CNS) depressants and antihistamines at the same time would produce:
   1. increased sedation.
   2. paradoxical excitation.
   3. urinary retention.
   4. tachycardia.

6. Evaluation of a patient with seasonal allergic rhinitis might reveal:
   1. cough productive of mucus.
   2. swollen, pale nasal passages and clear, watery nasal discharge.
   3. red, swollen nasal passages and thick, greenish discharge.
   4. musical or noisy sounds when the patient breathes in and out.

7. Antihistamines would be ordered by the physician for very young children:
   1. if the family has a history of sleep apnea
   2. if the child has symptoms of Reye's syndrome.
   3. cautiously, if at all.
   4. with one large dose at bedtime.

8. A 48-year-old patient at the clinic asks the nurse if she should be taking an antihistamine for her allergies because she also needs to be on aspirin for her arthritis. The best response would be:
   1. "You need to be careful taking an antihistamine along with aspirin because together they may cause hearing loss."
   2. "It is not safe to take these two medications together; you need to stop one of them."
   3. "You need to talk to your physician about the drug interactions."
   4. "Because these products are both available over the counter, they are safe together."

9. Patient teaching for antihistamine use for patients over the age of 65 needs to include which of the following? *(Select all that apply.)*
   1. These drugs are safe to take, because few bad reactions occur.
   2. These drugs may dry out your mouth and throat so drink lots of water along with them.
   3. Take with meals or milk to reduce any GI upset.
   4. Report any feelings of muscle stiffness, inability to walk, feelings of anxiety or restlessness, or strange new movements of your head, neck, or jaw to the physician.

10. Patients take antihistamines for which of the following reasons?
    1. help them sleep at night
    2. relieve symptoms of allergic reactions
    3. relieve symptoms of the common cold
    4. help them stay awake longer when tired

11. When the nurse talks to the patient about "rebound effect" with antihistamines, it means the appearance of original symptoms is caused by:
    1. long-term use of topical nasal antihistamines.
    2. taking antihistamines intramuscularly.
    3. an increased resistance to the drug.
    4. changing medications frequently.

12. Common side effects caused by antihistamines include: *(Select all that apply.)*
    1. GI upset.
    2. increased appetite.
    3. thickening of secretions.
    4. drowsiness.
    5. decreased sinus pressure.

PART II: ANTITUSSIVES

1. Antitussive agents are used to:
   1. promote expectoration (spitting of mucus).
   2. prevent a cough from developing.
   3. thin the secretions in the bronchial airways.
   4. relieve coughing.

2. Narcotic antitussives act by:
   1. Suppressing the desire of the patient to cough.
   2. Making the mucus very thick so it can be coughed up.
   3. Making patients sleepy so they don't cough.
   4. Suppressing or preventing the cough reflex by acting directly on the cough center in the brain.

3. Antitussive agents are used primarily in:
   1. patients who cannot sleep or work due to severe cough, mucus production, and fever.
   2. patients with a productive cough that is associated with pneumonia.
   3. nonproductive coughs.
   4. chronic allergic conditions.

4. The most common adverse reactions to antitussives include:
   1. drowsiness, dry mouth, and tachycardia.
   2. drowsiness, dry mouth, nausea, and postural hypotension.
   3. constipation; dry mouth; and dry, cracked mucosa.
   4. drowsiness, muscle aches, and high blood pressure.

5. A 72-year-old patient is being seen at the clinic for a chronic nonproductive cough. She has been given a narcotic antitussive to use. What precautions will the nurse instruct her about?
   1. "Do not operate heavy machinery or drink alcohol while taking the medication."
   2. "Drive the car only during the day; take your cough medicine only at night."
   3. "Alter the dose of the medication as your symptoms change."
   4. "If nausea occurs, stop taking the medication and call your health care provider."

6. For which of the following patients are antitussives contraindicated? *(Select all that apply.)*
   1. 78-year-old male with chronic obstructive pulmonary disease (COPD)
   2. 54-year-old male with an allergy to dextromethorphan
   3. 38-year-old female with diabetes
   4. 26-year-old female who is pregnant

7. Use the computer or a drug reference book to tell which of the following orders has the correct antitussive dose range for adults?
    1. Codeine 30 mg orally every 4 to 6 hours
    2. Tessalon Perles 100 mg orally three times daily
    3. Robitussin 40 mg orally every 4 hours
    4. Tusstat 50 mg orally every 4 hours

8. One of the most important points to teach a patient taking an antitussive medication would be:
    1. to take the medication as ordered by the health care provider.
    2. to drink lots of orange juice or water while taking this drug.
    3. that the medication may cause drowsiness or nausea.
    4. to take the drug with food or milk to decrease stomach upset.

PART III: MEDICATIONS USED IN THE TREATMENT OF ASTHMA AND COPD

1. What happens when the patient has a bronchospasm?
    1. More mucus is produced in the respiratory tract.
    2. Narrowing of the lumen restricts the amount of air that is pulled into or pushed out of the lungs with each breath.
    3. Vasodilation is produced.
    4. Bronchodilation results.

2. The two major types of bronchodilators are:
    1. theophylline and xanthines.
    2. sympathomimetics and adrenergics.
    3. sympathomimetics and xanthine derivatives.
    4. β_2 adrenergics and anticholinergics.

3. The major difference between asthma and COPD is:
    1. there is no difference. They are different words for the same problem.
    2. asthma is an acute illness, but COPD gets worse gradually over time.
    3. asthma gets worse over time, but COPD patients improve and become symptom-free.
    4. asthma is chronic and seldom symptom-free but COPD involves sudden attacks and worsening symptoms.

4. Sympathomimetics cause vasoconstriction in the blood vessels of the mucosa of the bronchi, which results in:
    1. reduction of edema in the mucosa and submucosal tissue of the respiratory tract.
    2. increased myocardial contractility.
    3. increased swelling and mucosal edema of the bronchi.
    4. increased mucus production and ciliary paralysis.

5. A 37-year-old female patient with a history of moderately severe asthma is complaining of not being hungry, feeling restless, and not being able to sleep at night. The nurse attributes her symptoms to:
    1. not enough bronchodilators which should help her sleep; dosage not sufficient.
    2. a common adverse reaction from her bronchodilators.
    3. a severe allergic reaction and a need to discontinue her medications at once.
    4. a need to educate her on the correct way to take her bronchodilators.

6. The patient is wheezing and complaining of shortness of breath. The nurse would expect the health care provider to order which to relieve bronchospasms?
    1. antitussives
    2. cromolyn sodium
    3. bronchodilators
    4. corticosteroids

7. When sympathomimetic bronchodilators appear to be ineffective, the patient might:
    1. use two different types of sympathomimetics at the same time.
    2. alternate two different sympathomimetic drugs.
    3. stop taking the medication, because an infection may be present.
    4. report the problem to the health care provider.

8. Refractoriness is:
    1. often caused by too-frequent use of drugs.
    2. infrequent with allergy and respiratory medications.
    3. caused when the underlying condition in the lung worsens.
    4. often related to food-drug interactions.

9. The main action of sympathomimetic bronchodilators is to:
   1. constrict the smooth muscles of the bron-
      chi.
   2. cause bronchial irritation.
   3. relax the smooth muscles of the bronchi so
      the lumen widens.
   4. increase the response caused by oxygen in
      the aerosol.

10. Mr. Allen complains that bronchodilators keep
    him from falling asleep at night. The nurse
    might suggest:
    1. taking the medication with a glass of warm
       milk at bedtime.
    2. taking a glass of alcohol to help him relax
       before going to bed.
    3. taking medication several hours before go-
       ing to bed.
    4. asking the health care provider for a mild
       sedative to counteract the effects of the
       bronchodilator.

11. The major difference in action between sympa-
    thomimetics and xanthine derivatives is that:
    1. xanthine derivatives produce significant
       CNS effects.
    2. xanthine derivatives act directly on smooth
       muscle to achieve bronchial constriction.
    3. xanthine derivatives do not have the sys-
       temic effects that sympathomimetics pro-
       duce.
    4. sympathomimetics also act directly on the
       kidneys to produce diuresis.

12. Aminophylline is an important agent to use to
    determine if the patient has bronchospasms or
    pulmonary edema. This agent is in the drug
    family of:
    1. sympathomimetic bronchodilators.
    2. leukotriene receptor inhibitors.
    3. xanthine bronchodilators.
    4. inhaled corticosteroids.

13. Chris is a 9-year-old boy who takes Theo-Dur
    regularly to control asthma symptoms. He has
    been playing in a soccer game today and came
    into the clinic because of constant coughing.
    The nurse finds that his pulse is irregular and
    determines that:
    1. vigorous exercise commonly causes an ir-
       regular pulse in children.
    2. overdosage with xanthine products often
       produces ventricular dysrhythmias.
    3. his symptoms probably indicate a need for
       increased medication.
    4. the exertion of playing soccer has caused
       the cardiac irregularity.

14. The half-life of xanthine bronchodilators is
    influenced by which of the following specific
    factors?
    1. age of the patient
    2. severity of the bronchospasm
    3. whether the patient smokes
    4. state of hydration of the patient

15. Monitoring the correct dosage of xanthine
    products is best accomplished by:
    1. decreasing the dose if the patient begins
       vomiting.
    2. determining if the use of prn medication is
       increasing.
    3. monitoring symptom relief.
    4. laboratory studies to measure the
       theophylline blood level.

16. Factors that affect the blood levels of theophyl-
    line include the: *(Select all that apply.)*
    1. age of the patient.
    2. varying theophylline-base in different
       products.
    3. metabolism and excretion of each drug.
    4. sex of the patient.

17. Patient teaching about the use of xanthine
    products includes: *(Select all that apply.)*
    1. reporting unusual symptoms like fast
       heartbeat, dizziness, and seizures.
    2. taking over-the-counter cough syrups with
       the xanthine product.
    3. if a dose is skipped and more than an hour
       has passed, stay on the original schedule.
    4. drinking a glass of water with the medica-
       tion and avoiding large amounts of caffein-
       ated drinks.

18. A 48-year-old female patient comes to the clinic complaining that she needs to urinate frequently after taking her asthma medication and is worried that she is getting diabetes. What can the nurse tell her?
    1. "Yes, it sounds like you are getting diabetes, we need to check your blood sugar."
    2. "No, it would be impossible for you to get diabetes at this age."
    3. "I believe that perhaps this is an effect of the medications you are on. Let's review them."
    4. "Have you had a bladder infection lately?"

19. Leukotriene receptor inhibitors are drugs that:
    1. control the severity of asthma.
    2. treat the acute attacks of asthma.
    3. prevent the exacerbations of COPD.
    4. reduce the symptoms of asthma.

20. Drugs that are known to interact with leukotriene receptor inhibitors include: (Select all that apply.)
    1. Tylenol.
    2. aspirin.
    3. Coumadin.
    4. theophylline.

21. The nurse is interviewing a patient who is to start on Singulair for chronic asthma. What questions are important to ask the patient? (Select all that apply.)
    1. "Are you currently pregnant or breastfeeding?" (to female patients)
    2. "Tell me how you would describe your current health."
    3. "Have you ever been told you have any liver disease?"
    4. "Tell me about your normal diet."

22. The patient has had asthma for years and takes several different medications for management. The treatment regimen has been changed to include corticosteroids, and the patient is anxious about the change. What will the nurse say to reassure him?
    1. "The addition of corticosteroids means your asthma is out of control and we need to treat it aggressively."
    2. "I wouldn't worry if I were you; the doctor knows what she's doing."
    3. "Corticosteroids are used for long-term asthma control and they help to prevent the airway getting smaller when exposed to an allergen (hyperresponsiveness)."
    4. "Corticosteroids are wonderful antiinflammatory drugs that are very safe."

23. Cromolyn sodium is a medication used for:
    1. acute treatment of severe asthma attacks.
    2. acute COPD relapse.
    3. prophylaxis of asthma attacks.
    4. acute treatment of exertional asthma.

24. Important patient teaching related to the use of cromolyn sodium includes: (Select all that apply.)
    1. "Take this drug every day at regular intervals."
    2. "Some patients get a cough after taking this drug; let us know if this happens."
    3. "Your symptoms should improve after 4 weeks."
    4. "You should be able to stop taking your other medications when this drug stabilizes your asthma."

25. Leukotriene receptor inhibitors are used primarily to:
    1. block bronchospasm.
    2. reduce inflammation.
    3. thin mucus secretions.
    4. dilate bronchioles.

26. Systemic corticosteroids are used primarily for the purpose of:
    1. boosting the action of cromolyn sodium.
    2. decreasing the inflammatory activity in the bronchioles.
    3. producing direct smooth muscle constriction.
    4. decreasing the effect of beta-adrenergic drugs.

27. Use of inhaled corticosteroids in asthma is for:
    1. severe episodes of asthma that do not respond to other drugs.
    2. short-term therapy only.
    3. solo drug therapy only.
    4. long-term control of symptoms.

PART IV: DECONGESTANTS

1. The nurse is giving instructions to a 34-year-old woman about the use of decongestants that are ordered for relief of pain from her ear infection. What are the points the nurse needs to cover? *(Select all that apply.)*
    1. "Make sure your children do not accidentally take any of this medication."
    2. "This should help relieve the pressure around your eustachian tubes caused from the ear infection."
    3. "This decongestant may cause some nervousness and nausea. If these symptoms do not improve after a time, let us know."
    4. "These are safe drugs to take and do not interfere with other medications."

2. If the patient has a viral cold, she would need:
    1. an expectorant to dry up her mucus.
    2. a decongestant to relieve nasal congestion.
    3. an antihistamine to stop his runny nose.
    4. both a decongestant and an antihistamine.

3. Decongestants are used for the relief of nasal congestion caused by: *(Select all that apply.)*
    1. ear infections.
    2. pneumonia.
    3. asthma.
    4. swollen lymph nodes.

4. When topical decongestants are used, which of the following can occur?
    1. hypotension
    2. dysrhythmias
    3. rebound congestion
    4. nervousness

5. The nurse understands that rebound congestion can lead to psychologic dependence and long-term use. What are ways to reduce the chance for dependence?
    1. Educate patients on the correct use of decongestants.
    2. Explain that oral decongestants are safer than topical.
    3. Refuse to allow patients to have decongestants.
    4. Warn patients that they must take the medication for at least 3 weeks or it won't be effective.

6. Decongestants are contraindicated in patients with all of the following conditions except:
    1. hypothyroidism.
    2. diabetes.
    3. hypertension.
    4. glaucoma.

7. A 27-year-old patient asks the nurse about the use of topical decongestants. The best response from the nurse is:
    1. "Tip your head back when using drops to avoid swallowing the drug."
    2. "Long-term use of topical decongestants is appropriate."
    3. "These decongestants are only available as sprays."
    4. "Use these topical preparations for 7-10 days so you can get a rebound effect."

8. An unpleasant side effect from nasal decongestants is:
    1. an increase in ear congestion.
    2. mild throat irritation.
    3. a burning and stinging of the nasal mucosa.
    4. a decrease in nasal drainage.

9. Go to the Internet or consult a drug reference book to decide which of the following orders should be questioned.
    1. oxymetazoline (Afrin) 2 squeezes each nostril twice daily
    2. phenylephrine (Sinex) 0.5% strength, 3-4 drops every 4 hours
    3. pseudoephedrine (Sudafed) 120 mg orally 3-4 times daily
    4. tetrahydrozoline (Tyzine) 2 drops each nostril every 4 hours

    Evaluate the Internet sites you visited. Which sites gave the best information? Did the sites all agree? Why or why not?

10. The patient asks the nurse which would be better—to take the topical decongestant or the oral one. The nurse's response would include:
    1. "It is always better to take the oral doses, as they are more effective."
    2. "I would suggest that you need to find out for yourself which one works best for you."
    3. "Topical decongestants are applied to the nasal mucosa and usually do not affect your whole system the way an oral preparation would."
    4. "Topical preparations can be used longer than oral preparations."

11. The nurse is teaching a patient on the proper way to instill nasal drops. Part of the instructions include: (*Select all that apply.*)
    1. "These solutions can become contaminated with bacteria, so be careful not to touch the skin when administering them."
    2. "Drops have a tendency to pass down your throat and get swallowed."
    3. "Topical administration helps the medication act on the nasal mucosa faster than if you took a pill."
    4. "Remember to tilt your head forward to allow the drops to flow back out of your nose."

PART V: EXPECTORANTS

1. It is thought that expectorants work in which way?
    1. They increase coughing which allows sputum to be expectorated (spit out).
    2. They increase the thickness of respiratory secretions.
    3. They decrease the thickness of respiratory secretions.
    4. They decrease the amount of water in the respiratory tract.

2. One of the major reasons expectorants are used is to relieve symptoms of:
    1. dry, nonproductive cough.
    2. loose, productive cough.
    3. irritating, dry cough.
    4. thick, productive cough.

3. Patient teaching instructions for a person using expectorants include: (*Select all that apply.*)
    1. "Using a humidifier is recommended in these cases."
    2. "You may find that it will make you cough more sputum."
    3. "If your cough returns once it has gone away, just start taking the drug again."
    4. "You will need to increase the amount of water you drink."

4. What will the nurse tell the patient with regard to side effects of expectorants?
    1. "You will need to drink more water with this medication."
    2. "The most common reaction people get is some GI upset."
    3. "The medication will make you cough more."
    4. "You should take the medication every 4 hours."

5. It is recommended that patients who are also taking anticoagulants not take which expectorant?
    1. Robitussin
    2. SSKI
    3. Mucinex
    4. Iophen R-Gen

6. Which expectorant must not be used continuously because it may lead to hypothyroidism?
    1. Robitussin
    2. SSKI
    3. Mucinex
    4. Iophen R-Gen

7. Expectorants work best when patients who take them also increase their:
    1. fluid intake.
    2. exercise time.
    3. coughing.
    4. sleep time.

PART VI: INTRANASAL STEROIDS

1. The main action of intranasal steroids is:
    1. increasing the local blood supply in the nasal mucosa.
    2. stimulation of the inflammatory response.
    3. beta-stimulation of adrenergic receptors.
    4. suppression of the inflammatory reaction.

2. Topical intranasal steroids are used in the treatment of which of the following conditions? *(Select all that apply.)*
   1. allergic symptoms
   2. inflammation from nasal polyps
   3. inflammation from irritating chemicals
   4. loss of the ability to smell

3. The patient has just been started on intranasal steroids and she asks the nurse if there are any possible drug interactions. The nurse replies:
   1. "No, they are safe to take."
   2. "I can check for you using the list of medications you are taking."
   3. "These medications are only of concern when you get an infection."
   4. "They only interact with other inhaled medications."

4. Some adverse reactions to be aware of while taking intranasal steroids which would require stopping the medication include:
   1. cracked or bleeding nasal mucosa.
   2. increased blood pressure, weight gain.
   3. weight loss, anorexia.
   4. lightheadedness, flashing lights before eyes.

5. Steroids pose a risk in their use because the drug may increase the risk for:
   1. infections.
   2. hearing loss.
   3. dependency.
   4. asthma.

6. Which of the following conditions are contraindicated for intranasal steroid use? *(Select all that apply.)*
   1. pregnancy
   2. asthma
   3. herpes infection of the lip
   4. infections of the lung

7. Identify the class of drugs for the following medications:

   1. _____ Decongestants
   2. _____ Antihistamines
   3. _____ Intranasal steroids
   4. _____ Leukotriene receptor antagonists
   5. _____ Antitussives
   6. _____ Expectorants
   7. _____ Long-acting B_2-adrenergic agonist bronchodilators
   8. _____ Corticosteroids

   a. fluticasone (Flovent)
   b. albuterol (Proventil)
   c. beclomethasone (Beclovent)
   d. pseudoephedrine (Sudafed)
   e. Certrizine (Zyrtec)
   f. loratadine (Claritin)
   g. diphenhydramine (Benadryl)
   h. theophylline (Slo-Phyllin)
   i. salmeterol (Serevent)
   j. phenylephrine (Neo-Synephrine)
   k. triamcinolone (Nasacort)
   l. cromolyn (NasalCrom)
   m. guaifenesin (Robitussin)
   n. dextromethorphan (Delsym)
   o. montelukast
   p. prednisone

PART VII: MASTERING ALLERGY AND RESPIRATORY MEDICATIONS

1. Talk with your friends or ask your school to find a canister that has been used for delivery of a corticosteroid to the lungs such as used in asthma. If you were given this canister by a pharmacist, what questions would you ask? What would you want to know? When do you put the canister in your nose and when do you put the canister to your lips?

   Go to the Internet and find out how you are supposed to use the canister if you are to prevent an asthma attack. Why wouldn't you want to use this type of medication if you were already having an asthma attack? How do you know when the canister is empty?

2. Everyone has had a runny nose and a cough. Talk with your class members about your experiences. What medications have you taken? Did you have any adverse effects from any of these medications? Were they helpful? Have you learned anything in this pharmacology class that would have changed any medicines that you took or anything that you did?

3. Asthma and COPD produce very different breathing problems. Do you know anyone who has these problems? When you look at people with these problems, do people with asthma look different than people with COPD? Ask them about the medicines they take and if they are helpful or not. Have they had adverse effects from any of their medications?

Antiinfective Medications

chapter

9

e Go to http://evolve.elsevier.com/edmunds/lpn/ for additional activities and exercises.

PART I: PENICILLINS

1. The most common signs of infection include:
   1. joint stiffness, pain on movement.
   2. nausea, heartburn, feeling of fullness.
   3. headache, sore throat, coughing, stuffy nose.
   4. redness, swelling, pain, fever.

2. The term for an antiinfective or antimicrobial drug that is effective for a large number of organisms is:
   1. narrow-spectrum.
   2. broad-spectrum.
   3. bacteriostatic.
   4. bactericidal.

3. You are caring for an 18-year-old woman who has been admitted to the hospital with a high temperature and cough. She has been diagnosed with pneumococcal pneumonia and oral amoxicillin has been ordered. Things you will want to teach the patient include: (Select all that apply.)
   1. take all of the medication; every dose should be taken.
   2. notify your health care provider if you develop a rash, hives, or trouble breathing.
   3. penicillin will interfere with any oral contraceptives you may be taking; use a second form of birth control other than oral contraceptives while you are taking the antibiotic.
   4. photosensitivity will develop; you need to stay indoors.

4. Your 48-year-old patient has just been diagnosed with neuropathy from taking penicillin for treatment of bacterial endocarditis. He asks you what "neuropathy" means. Your best response would be:
   1. "I think it has something to do with your kidneys."
   2. "The drug you were on caused some damage to your muscles."
   3. "It is an adverse reaction from penicillin that has caused nerve damage."
   4. "It means you have a superinfection."

5. The patient tells you she is allergic to penicillin because she has nausea and vomiting every time she has taken it. You would explain:
   1. "It is not a real allergic reaction unless you stop breathing."
   2. "You only have an allergic reaction if you have problems with the first dose."
   3. "It is not an allergic reaction unless you also have rash, itching, and diarrhea."
   4. "Nausea and vomiting are likely a common side effect and not an allergy."

6. Widespread use of penicillin has led to which of the following problems? (Select all that apply.)
   1. penicillin-resistant organisms
   2. pathogenic organisms
   3. superinfections
   4. narrow-spectrum drugs

7.   Match the common infection with the causative organism.

Infection		Causative Organism	
1. _____	strep throat	a.	*Corynebacterium diphtheriae*
2. _____	meningitis	b.	*Clostridium tetani*
3. _____	diphtheria	c.	*Neisseria gonorrhoeae*
4. _____	impetigo	d.	*Neisseria meningitidis*
5. _____	tetanus	e.	beta-hemolytic streptococci
6. _____	syphilis	f.	*Treponema pallidum*
7. _____	gonorrhea	g.	Staphylococcus

PART II: SULFONAMIDES

1.   Infections that require the use of sulfonamides include: *(Select all that apply.)*
    1.   cystitis.
    2.   stomatitis.
    3.   acute otitis media.
    4.   hepatitis

2.   You are caring for a 63-year-old female patient who is being treated with sulfonamides for conjunctivitis. She asks if it is still okay to take Dyazide for her high blood pressure. Your response would include:
    1.   "It should be fine to take your other medications."
    2.   "The effect of Dyazide may be increased with the use of this sulfa drug."
    3.   "Some people are hypersensitive to sulfonamides, but you should not be because you do not have any allergies."
    4.   "The effect of Dyazide may be decreased with the use of this sulfa drug."

3.   What special instructions should you include in your teaching for patients taking sulfonamides?
    1.   "You will need to drink large amounts of water with this drug to prevent urinary stones."
    2.   "You should take this drug on an empty stomach, because food will deactivate it."
    3.   "You should be able to continue your normal outdoor activities."
    4.   "You may get some vertigo and tinnitus with this drug."

4.   Sulfonamides are:
    1.   relatively new drugs.
    2.   very hard on the stomach and may cause ulcers.
    3.   produce traveler's diarrhea.
    4.   contraindicated if the patient is pregnant.

5.   Which lab tests are important to be done prior to starting on sulfonamides? *(Select all that apply.)*
    1.   kidney function tests: creatinine, BUN
    2.   urinalysis
    3.   albumin level
    4.   complete blood count

6.   Some potentially serious adverse reactions for which the nurse and patient must watch for include: *(Select all that apply.)*
    1.   photosensitivity.
    2.   blood dyscrasias.
    3.   anaphylactic shock.
    4.   toxemia.

7. Use your textbook to determine the drug interaction that use of these medications would have with a sulfonamide product by placing an "X" in the corresponding box.

Medication	Increase effect of drug	Decrease effect of drug	Decrease absorption of sulfonamide	Increase effect of sulfonamide
Oral anticoagulants				
Probenecid				
Thiazide diuretics				
Salicylates				
Indomethacin				
Penicillin				
Antacids				
Phenytoin				
Uricosuric agents				

8. Your patient asks you what is meant by the term *stomatitis*. Your response would be:
   1. "Stomatitis is an infection in your stomach."
   2. "Stomatitis is an adverse reaction that will cause you to itch very badly."
   3. "Stomatitis is an inflammation of the mouth."
   4. "Stomatitis is just a fancy word for low blood sugar."

9. *Tinnitus* refers to:
   1. drowsiness and fatigue.
   2. feeling of dizziness.
   3. ringing in the ears.
   4. lack of appetite.

10. The development of proteinuria, hematuria, and crystalluria can be avoided by giving which of the following instructions to patients taking sulfonamides?
    1. "Get a good night's sleep."
    2. "Take the medication on an empty stomach."
    3. "Avoid the sun."
    4. "Drink plenty of water with the medication."

11. Sulfonamide products can be used for which of the following infections? *(Select all that apply.)*
    1. ocular infections
    2. vaginal infections
    3. urinary tract infections
    4. skin infections

12. *Prophylactic* use of antibiotics means the use of antibiotics to prevent:
    1. infections.
    2. superinfections.
    3. otitis media.
    4. dyscrasias.

PART III: BROAD-SPECTRUM ANTIBIOTICS

1. Broad-spectrum antibiotics:
   1. are relatively new products on the market.
   2. are effective against viral, parasitic, or fungal infections.
   3. do not often cause serious adverse effects and so are seen as the safest drugs on the market.
   4. are effective against both gram-positive and gram-negative organisms.

2. *Bacteriostatic* refers to the ability of the antiinfective to:
   1. kill the bacteria.
   2. slow the growth of the bacteria.
   3. attack the internal cell processes.
   4. destroy the external cell walls.

3. The term *mixed infection* refers to:
   1. one infection following another.
   2. more than one infection occurring at the same time.
   3. an overgrowth of organisms.
   4. mild infection with the diagnosis is not clear.

4. The use of an appropriate antiinfective is determined by the: *(Select all that apply.)*
   1. culture and sensitivity of the organism.
   2. the antibiotic most effective against the organism.
   3. cheapest one available.
   4. classification of organism as gram-positive or gram-negative.

5. Your patient asks what the doctor meant when she told him that he has a *gram-negative* infection. Your response would be:
   1. "That means that the organism that you have stains positive when the laboratory checks it."
   2. "That means that the organism that is causing your infection has become resistant to other antibiotics."
   3. "That mean that the organism that you have is negative when the lab checks it."
   4. "That means that the results of the laboratory test were negative."

6. Broad-spectrum antiinfectives are used for which types of infections?
   1. viral
   2. parasitic
   3. fungal
   4. bacterial

7. The three types of major adverse reactions seen with antibiotic therapy include:
   1. superinfections, hepatotoxicity, allergic reactions.
   2. allergic reactions, cross-sensitivity, GI irritations.
   3. ototoxicity, GI irritations, allergic reactions.
   4. allergic reactions, secondary infections, mixed infections.

8. Superinfections are commonly caused by:
   1. GI irritation.
   2. allergic reactions.
   3. long-term use of antibiotics.
   4. use of broad-spectrum antibiotics.

9. Tissue damage that may occur from antibiotics may affect several organs such as: *(Select all that apply.)*
   1. liver—hepatotoxicity.
   2. ear—ototoxicity.
   3. GI—toxicity.
   4. kidney—nephrotoxicity.

10. Some antibiotics cause symptoms specific to an injured body part; other symptoms affect the body in general. What would be an example of a symptom specific to an injured body part? *(Select all that apply.)*
    1. nausea, vomiting, and diarrhea
    2. ringing in the ears and hearing loss
    3. decrease in urine output
    4. general malaise, elevated liver enzymes, jaundiced skin

11. Your patient has a history of many drug allergies and is concerned about developing an allergy to the antibiotic ordered for his urinary tract infection. You will reassure him, answer questions, and tell him:
    1. "The possibility of developing another allergy is very small, don't worry about it."
    2. "The hypersensitivity reactions that we see in the clinic are very rare."
    3. "The people most likely to develop a drug allergy are people who have a history of drug allergies."
    4. "The number of times I have seen cross-sensitivity to antibiotics I could count on one hand."

12. Mild allergic reactions might include: *(Select all that apply.)*
    1. skin rash.
    2. cross-sensitivity.
    3. fever.
    4. laryngeal edema.

13. Anaphylaxis is the most serious form of hypersensitivity and may be shown by:
    1. shortness of breath, laryngeal edema, shock.
    2. drowsiness, skin rash, nausea.
    3. shortness of breath, vomiting, hepatotoxicity.
    4. drowsiness, ototoxicity, diarrhea.

14. If a patient is allergic to penicillin, the drug of choice is often:
    1. sulfonamides.
    2. cephalosporins.
    3. aminoglycosides.
    4. lincosamides.

15. The antiinfective cefaclor (Ceclor) is considered a:
    1. first-generation cephalosporin.
    2. second-generation cephalosporin.
    3. third-generation cephalosporin.
    4. fourth-generation cephalosporin.

16. Symptoms of bone marrow depression caused by the use of antiinfectives include:
    1. increased blood sugar, malaise, jaundice.
    2. decreased urine output, fever, skin rash.
    3. bruising, petechiae, sore throat.
    4. nausea, vomiting, diarrhea.

17. In the following table, identify for each specific antibiotic the most important adverse reaction to monitor by placing an "X" in the box corresponding to the reaction.

Antibiotic	Severe GI Upset	Nephrotoxicity	Fatal Colitis
clindamycin			
colistin			
erythromycin			
aminoglycosides			
lincomycin			

18. The difference between oral and parenteral antibiotics is that oral antibiotics are:
    1. safer, whereas parenteral antibiotics should be used with caution.
    2. cheaper, whereas parenteral antibiotics are more expensive.
    3. to be avoided, whereas parenteral antibiotics are better tolerated.
    4. to be used with caution, whereas parenteral antibiotics are safer.

19. The effect of gastrointestinal upset can be managed if the oral antibiotics are:
    1. given with food.
    2. taken on an empty stomach.
    3. fully chewed before swallowing.
    4. swallowed with minimal water.

20. Your patient says the health care provider started him on a *third-generation* antibiotic. He asks you, "What does that mean?" Your best response would be:
    1. "The third-generation drugs are cousins of the original antibiotics like penicillin."
    2. "The third-generation antibiotics are more effective against resistant organisms."
    3. "The first-generation antibiotics don't work anymore, so we have to use the more effective third generation."
    4. "I don't know. I think it means the latest drug on the market but ask your doctor."

21. There are many drugs to remember. Look at the drug lists in the book. Are there any hints in the way the drugs are named that helps you remember to which drug category they belong? Are there key words, symbols, images, rhymes, or other things that can help you remember some of the names? (for example: "Lincomycin helps link the really powerful dangerous organism to the drug.")

22. Several places in the book the nurse is told that a patient having an anaphylactic reaction will have laryngeal edema. What is laryngeal edema and how will the nurse know if the patient is having this? Go to your nursing textbooks or the Internet to answer this question.

23. Some medications, including some antibiotics, may cause bone marrow depression. What does this mean and how would you suspect this is happening? Go to your nursing textbooks or the Internet to answer this question.

24. While some specific medications may cause adverse effects (for example, tetracycline given to young children will permanently stain their teeth a dark color), the nurse should always be observing the patient for any unusual symptoms that might suggest a serious adverse effect is occurring. Go to your nursing textbooks or the Internet and learn what symptoms would be present in the following common but serious adverse effects:

Adverse reaction	Symptoms
Renal toxicity	
Hepatotoxicity	
Ototoxicity	
Ocular effects	
Neurotoxicity	

25. What is an idiosyncratic drug reaction? How would you find out if the strange symptoms your patient is reporting are normal for the medications he is taking, or something new?

PART IV: ANTITUBERCULAR AGENTS

1. The persons most likely to be infected with tuberculosis are: *(Select all that apply.)*
   1. drug users.
   2. AIDS patients.
   3. immigrants from South America.
   4. immigrants from Europe.

2. Several different drugs are used at the same time to treat tuberculosis for which reason?
   1. The bacterium has a very hard cell wall.
   2. They slow the development of bacterial resistance to the drugs.
   3. Because of the expense of the medications.
   4. Because of the toxicity of the combination drugs.

3. Tuberculosis is a disease that requires new guidelines every year from which organization?
   1. MDR
   2. CDC
   3. PZA
   4. INH

4. Antituberculosis therapy that does not kill the bacterium but prevents its spread through the patient or to other individuals is known as:
   1. chemoprophylaxis.
   2. chemotherapy.
   3. bacteriostatic.
   4. bactericidal.

5. Drug resistance is likely to develop when what occurs?
   1. patient compliance
   2. active hepatitis
   3. only one drug is used
   4. the culture converts to negative

6. The term *antitubercular chemoprophylaxis* refers to:
   1. weight loss associated with antitubercular drugs.
   2. the use of drugs to treat a disease.
   3. the use of drugs to prevent a disease.
   4. psychologic changes or changes in personality.

7. Many of the medications used to treat tuberculosis are associated with severe tissue damage to the:
   1. kidneys and nerves.
   2. brain and spinal cord.
   3. liver and pancreas.
   4. bones and muscles.

8. The difference between primary and secondary agents used for treatment of tuberculosis is that primary agents are:
   1. cheaper than secondary agents.
   2. more effective than secondary agents.
   3. more toxic than secondary agents.
   4. used for more drug-resistant organisms than secondary agents.

9. In which organs can antitubercular drugs cause toxicity? *(Select all that apply.)*
   1. lungs
   2. liver
   3. kidneys
   4. ears

10. Use a drug reference book to determine which of the following drug orders is accurate.
    1. isoniazid 600 mg orally daily
    2. rifampin 600 mg orally daily
    3. rifapentine 150 mg orally daily
    4. ethambutol 15 mg orally daily

    Which are the best drug reference books to use to find this answer?

11. Active tuberculosis infection symptoms include: *(Select all that apply.)*
    1. night sweats.
    2. increased appetite.
    3. productive cough.
    4. weight gain.
    5. fever.

12. You are taking care of a 68-year-old male patient who asks you what he should do if he misses a dose of his TB drugs. Your response should include:
    1. "You should take the dose as soon as you remember."
    2. "You will have to skip the dose and take a double dose the next day."
    3. "You will need to notify the physician if you skip a dose."
    4. "You will have to come in for more lab tests if you miss a dose."

13. General characteristics of antitubercular therapy for active tuberculosis include: *(Select all that apply.)*
    1. giving one drug for active tuberculosis.
    2. giving several drugs for active tuberculosis.
    3. short-term drug therapy.
    4. long-term drug therapy.
    5. multiple dosing during the day.
    6. one-time daily dosing.
    7. parenteral medication only.
    8. oral medication only.

14. Most antitubercular medications cause gastric irritation and should be taken with food. Identify the one medication that is better absorbed on an empty stomach.
    1. rifampin
    2. isoniazid
    3. pyrazinamide
    4. ethambutol

15. The discharge instructions to a patient who is being treated for TB include: *(Select all that apply.)*
    1. "You will need to get a Medic-Alert bracelet."
    2. "You will need to be monitored frequently with lab tests to make sure that these drugs are working."
    3. "You will need to have your entire family treated for TB."
    4. "You will need to report adverse reactions promptly."
    5. "You will need to follow the directions for taking your medications exactly."
    6. "You will need to dispose of soiled tissues carefully."

16. If a patient has been treated for tuberculosis previously and becomes symptomatic again, what should be suspected?
    1. HIV infection
    2. patient compliance issues
    3. culture conversion to negative
    4. drug interactions

17. Use of ethambutol may lead to the development of:
    1. drug resistance.
    2. ototoxicity.
    3. narrow therapeutic range.
    4. psychologic changes.

18. Monitoring of treatment effectiveness of antitubercular drugs includes:
    1. patient's weight.
    2. blood level of the antibiotic.
    3. BUN and creatinine levels.
    4. culture and sensitivity.

19. In the following table, identify for each specific antitubercular drug the most important adverse reaction to monitor by placing an "X" in the box corresponding to the reaction. *(More than one may apply.)*

Antitubercular drug	Headache	Drowsiness	Paresthesia	Dizziness	Vision disturbances	Ototoxicity
Isoniazid						
Streptomycin sulfate						
Rifampin						
Capreomycin						
Ethambutol						

20. Why do we spend so much time talking about tuberculosis? This is a disease that was a frequent cause of death before antibiotics were developed. Now we have many drugs to treat it. Do some reading about tuberculosis. Who is at risk for developing tuberculosis? Are you as a nurse at risk for TB?

21. Go to the Internet to learn about ways that different states make sure patients with TB take their medications. Some of the methods affect patients; some of the methods also are for health care providers. Why do states worry about whether patients take their TB medications or not?

PART V: ANTIPARASITIC AGENTS

1. What parasite causes amebiasis?
   1. *Plasmodium falciparum*
   2. *Entamoeba histolytica*
   3. *Trichomonas vaginalis*
   4. *Chlamydia trachomatis*

2. What is meant by an *extraintestinal* infection?
   1. ulcerative colitis
   2. infection in the heart, such as bacterial endocarditis
   3. infection outside of the GI tract, such as hepatic abscess
   4. urticarial rash

3. What are two of the major drugs used for the treatment of amebiasis?
   1. metronidazole and paromomycin
   2. diiodohydroxyquin and ampicillin
   3. chloroquine and ticarcillin
   4. paromomycin and gentamicin

4. The common precautions or contraindications for the use of amebicides include: *(Select all that apply.)*
   1. take all drugs as prescribed.
   2. side effects are very common.
   3. take the drug for up to 1 year.
   4. wash hands after going to the bathroom.
   5. take the drug with food to reduce stomach upset.

5. Identify the one amebicide known to cause poor coordination.
   1. metronidazole
   2. paromomycin
   3. diiodohydroxyquin
   4. chloroquine

6. Parasites are invading organisms that include which of the following? *(Select all that apply.)*
   1. amoebas
   2. protozoans
   3. helminths
   4. viruses

7. Selection of the appropriate anthelmintic must be based on: *(Select all that apply.)*
   1. type of worm present.
   2. effectiveness of the drug.
   3. ability of the patient to be compliant.
   4. presence of hypertension.

8. Indicate the drug of choice for different types of worms by putting an "X" in the corresponding box.

Anthelmintic	Pinworms	Roundworms	Hookworms	Tapeworms
Pyrantel				
Piperazine				
Mebendazole				
Thiabendazole				
Niclosamide				

9. Once the type of worm is identified, special instructions should be given to the patient about how to avoid spreading the infestation. These instructions include:
   1. "It may be necessary to boil your sheets twice a day for several weeks."
   2. "It is easy to pass on the infection; all your family members must be treated as well."
   3. "You urine may develop an asparagus-like odor from the drugs."
   4. "You will become anemic, so taking iron supplements is recommended."

10. The people most susceptible to getting malaria include those: *(Select all that apply.)*
    1. traveling to areas that have malaria.
    2. who do not wash their hands after using the bathroom.
    3. eating raw foods without washing them first.
    4. who are bitten by a mosquito.
    5. who work as migrant farmers.

11. What happens when a mosquito infected with malaria bites a person? The protozoan travels from the blood to the:
    1. stomach where it reproduces.
    2. muscles where it reproduces.
    3. salivary glands where it reproduces.
    4. red blood cells where it reproduces.

12. Which protozoan causes malaria?
    1. Plasmodium
    2. Trichomonas
    3. Entamoeba
    4. Treponema

13. Why are a variety of medications used in the treatment of malaria?
    1. Not all drugs are effective against all four species of Plasmodium.
    2. Many strains of Plasmodium have developed resistance.
    3. The antimalarial drugs suppress the infection but often do not cure it.
    4. Some of the drugs are specific for extraintestinal infections.

14. Antimalarial preparations are used for:
    1. preventing malaria.
    2. treating the symptoms of malaria.
    3. infections caused by *Plasmodium falciparum*.
    4. suppressing and treating acute malaria attacks.

15. *Cinchonism* is another name for:
    1. atrophic glossitis.
    2. quinine poisoning.
    3. blood dyscrasias.
    4. malaria attacks.

16. The symptoms of cinchonism include:
    1. dizziness and diarrhea.
    2. fever and restlessness.
    3. nausea and headache.
    4. tinnitus and visual blurring.

17. The use of any antimalarial drugs can cause which of the following symptoms?
    1. ototoxicity
    2. cardiac dysrhythmias
    3. nephrotoxicity
    4. psychological changes

18. Symptoms of malaria include: *(Select all that apply.)*
    1. restlessness.
    2. periods of fever and chills.
    3. headache and nausea.
    4. profound sweating.

PART VI: MASTERING ANTIINFECTIVE MEDICATION CONCEPTS

1. How do organisms develop resistance to antibiotics? Go to the Internet and read about antibiotic resistance. How serious a problem is antibiotic resistance? Is this a local problem, a state problem, a national problem, or an international problem? What is predicted in the future about drug resistance? What new medications are being developed to solve this problem? As a class, discuss what principles are essential to slowing the development of drug-resistant organisms?

2. You notice on television that an advertisement by a pharmaceutical company suggests that patients should ask their doctors to give them a particular antibiotic. What do you think about this type of advertising directly to the patient? Does this type of advertising have any effect on the behavior of patients when they are sick?

3. Are there any conditions for which patients have to take antibiotics for years? What kinds of problems might these patients experience?

4. Some communities have a problem with methicillin-resistant *Staphylococcus aureus* infections. What does this mean? Which people in the community often get sick with this illness and what can be done to prevent it?

Antivirals, Antiretrovirals, and Antifungal Medications

chapter **10**

Go to http://evolve.elsevier.com/edmunds/lpn/ for additional activities and exercises.

PART I: ANTIVIRAL AND ANTIRETROVIRAL MEDICATIONS

1. Why do you think that LPN/LVNs need to know about medications for HIV?

2. Retroviruses are:
   1. messenger RNA that codes for HIV polyprotein.
   2. viruses that contain RNA and DNA.
   3. viruses that contain only DNA.
   4. cellular assembly units inside the lymphocytes.

3. The way drugs can combat the HIV infection include: *(Fill in the blanks.)*

   1. _____ the binding of HIV to DC4 receptors.

   2. Reverse transcriptase inhibitors prevent the HIV enzyme reverse transcriptase from _____.

   3. _____ with the viral assembly.

   4. _____ cellular mechanism to copy its RNA.

4. The types of drugs used to treat HIV and AIDS include: *(Select all that apply.)*
   1. antiviral medications.
   2. antifungal medications.
   3. reverse transcriptase inhibitors.
   4. antiretroviral medications.

5. Viral infections that may be treated by medications include:
   1. pancreatitis, hepatitis.
   2. appendicitis, gallbladder infection.
   3. mumps, measles, diphtheria.
   4. herpes simplex, herpes zoster, influenza A.

6. The nurse is instructing a 34-year-old male patient on taking his antiretroviral drugs. The most important thing to stress is:
   1. "You will have to let your health care provider know if you start to develop any numbness or burning in your fingers."
   2. "You need to take this medication for a limited time only because this will cure the infection in 10 days."
   3. "You need to be cautious about taking over-the-counter medications and let your health care provider know if you use them, because they may interfere with your prescription medications."
   4. "You will need to come in to see your health care provider if you get a sore throat and dry cough."

7. The two types of antiretroviral medications that LPN/LVNs may commonly give include:
   1. reverse transcriptase inhibitors and antibiotics.
   2. antivirals and protease inhibitors.
   3. antivirals and antifungals.
   4. protease inhibitors and reverse transcriptase inhibitors.

8. The nurse understands that despite taking medication, AIDS-related opportunistic infections develop because the:
   1. opportunistic infections damage the body's immune system.
   2. retrovirus damages the body's immune system.
   3. infections cause damage to the liver.
   4. infections cause damage to the P-450 cytochrome system.

9. The nurse knows that effectiveness of the medications is monitored through which laboratory tests?
   1. CD4 count, WBC count, liver function tests
   2. liver enzymes, blood clotting time
   3. blood culture and sensitivity
   4. cytochrome P-450 levels of liver

10. *Crix belly* refers to the development of:
    1. a large cyst on the leg and decreased plasma glucose.
    2. elevated triglycerides and accumulated fat in the abdomen.
    3. weight loss and increased plasma glucose.
    4. elevated triglycerides and accumulated fat in the arms and legs.

11. The nurse needs to know about and recognize Crix belly because:
    1. it will develop in all patients who are taking HIV medications.
    2. it represents a serious side effect of medication.
    3. this means that the medications are not working.
    4. this problem will require hospitalization.

PART II: ANTIFUNGAL MEDICATIONS

1. A *mycotic infection* refers to an infection that is caused by:
   1. reverse transcriptase inhibitors.
   2. pancreatitis.
   3. yeastlike organisms.
   4. a mycosis.

2. Fungi requiring medication treatment are found in which two major places in the body?
   1. the liver and the immune system
   2. the lungs and the nailbeds and skin
   3. the kidneys and the central nervous system
   4. the liver and the endocrine system

3. Antifungal medications may be sold by prescription or over the counter. The more commonly used antifungal medications include:
   1. nystatin, ketoconazole, amphotericin B, cidofovir.
   2. acyclovir, ketoconazole, griseofulvin, efavirenz.
   3. flucytosine, nystatin, griseofulvin, ketoconazole.
   4. metronidazole, ketoconazole, nystatin, nelfinavir.

4. What is the name of the organism that frequently causes vaginal infections in women and that is now seen so commonly in AIDS patients?
   1. Cryptococcus
   2. Candida
   3. Microsporum
   4. Trichophyton

5. An adverse drug reaction associated with antifungal medications is:
   1. hepatotoxicity.
   2. rare.
   3. generally mild, transient, and dosage-related.
   4. generally irritating but not very serious.

6. Superinfections, especially in immunocompromised patients, may result with prolonged use of antifungals concurrently with:
   1. antacids.
   2. anticholinergics.
   3. corticosteroids.
   4. H_2 blockers.

7. Antifungal medication can be delivered by which route(s)? *(Select all that apply.)*
   1. topically
   2. orally
   3. rectally
   4. vaginally

8. Antifungal medications have which of the following actions? *(Select all that apply.)*
   1. Allow intracellular components to leak through the cell membrane.
   2. Increase cell membrane permeability.
   3. Inhibit nucleic acid synthesis.
   4. Suppress reverse transcriptase.

PART III: MASTERING ANTIVIRALS, ANTIRETROVIRALS, AND ANTIFUNGAL MEDICATIONS

1. Go to the Internet and find out information about the drugs used to treat HIV infection. Share with your classmates where you found the best sources of information and why you think it was the best. Which sources do you believe are the more reliable and unbiased?

2. What kind of risk do you as a nurse have in working with patients who are HIV-positive? How can you protect yourself from infection? Are there guidelines that hospital employees must follow in working with HIV-positive patients? If you stuck your finger with a needle just taken from a patient who was HIV-positive, what would you do?

Antineoplastic Medications

e Go to http://evolve.elsevier.com/edmunds/lpn/ for additional activities and exercises.

PART I: ANTINEOPLASTIC AGENTS

1. You are caring for a 48-year-old female patient diagnosed with breast cancer, who asks you what to expect from the cyclophosphamide (Cytoxan) that the physician ordered. Your response would include: *(Select all that apply.)*
   1. "You will have nausea, vomiting, anorexia, and diarrhea with almost all your drugs, so we will be proactive and try to reduce these effects."
   2. "We want to reduce the urge you have to vomit, so we will restrict the amount of water you drink."
   3. "You will have to stay in the hospital the whole time so we can manage your side effects."
   4. "You will not have to worry about losing your hair; these drugs do not have that effect."

2. Antiemetics are used to control the symptom of:
   1. diarrhea.
   2. alopecia.
   3. nausea.
   4. anorexia.

3. What is the common side effect involving the mouth when antineoplastic agents are administered?
   1. stomatitis
   2. diarrhea
   3. pruritus
   4. gynecomastia

4. Drug orders for antineoplastic therapy may be different than you usually see. Most antineoplastic drug therapy is given by physicians only and calculated in milligrams per:
   1. pound.
   2. kilogram.
   3. ounce.
   4. milliliter.

5. Some antineoplastic medications cause bone marrow depression, which may cause:
   1. alopecia and anorexia.
   2. ocular effects and hypersensitivity.
   3. bleeding and bruising.
   4. nausea and vomiting.

6. What is the effect on the cells of the bone marrow when antineoplastic agents are administered?
   1. hypersensitivity to these drugs, causing skin eruptions
   2. anorexia, causing weight loss
   3. weakening the immune system and increasing risk of infections
   4. renal toxicity, causing a buildup of the drugs in blood instead of excretion

7. You are caring for a 67-year-old male patient diagnosed with leukemia. He says he is taking drugs to prevent metastasis, but he doesn't know what that means. Your response would be:
   1. "I think that you need to ask your doctor that question. I am responsible for giving you your medications."
   2. "When abnormal cells start growing at an unusually fast rate, they can invade other parts of the body."
   3. "It seems that metastasis happens when someone has leukemia, so it is just a fancy term we use."
   4. "Metastasis refers to the way the drugs work that we give you for treating your leukemia."

8. Because patients with malignancies are often so fearful about the unknown, it is important to remember that when they take medications:
   1. there is very little chance therapy will be helpful.
   2. the patient can be taught more information about their problem and their therapy.
   3. it is important for the nurse to conceal any bad news from the patient.
   4. medications are often helpful only when given intravenously as soon as the patient is diagnosed.

9. What is frequently the effect on ovaries or testes when antineoplastic agents are administered?
   1. Infertility may develop.
   2. Alopecia may happen.
   3. Anorexia always happens.
   4. Nausea always happens.

10. From the list below, circle all the cells that are naturally fast-growing, and thus likely to be affected by antineoplastic agents.

hair follicles	lining of the mouth
lining of the bladder	lining of the GI tract
bone marrow	nervous system
hepatocytes (liver cells)	

11. Antineoplastic or chemotherapeutic agents are used to treat:
    1. side effects.
    2. malignant diseases.
    3. alopecia.
    4. renal toxicity.

12. What is the most common side effect on the GI tract when antineoplastic agents are administered?
    1. runny nose
    2. alopecia
    3. diarrhea
    4. constipation

13. **Challenge Activity:** Match the action of the antineoplastic drug with the effect by placing an "X" in the box corresponding with the correct effect.

Antineoplastic drug type	Interferes with normal cell division	Interferes with various metabolic functions	Counteracts effects of tumors dependent on estrogens or testosterone	Stops cell division directly	Interferes with DNA and RNA synthesis
alkylating agents					
antimetabolites					
antibiotics					
hormones					
mitotic inhibitors					

PART II: MASTERING ANTINEOPLASTIC MEDICATIONS

1. Antineoplastic medications are very toxic and usually given by specialist physicians. Why should LPN/LVNs learn about these drugs? Discuss this with your classmates.

2. Many patients with cancer are worried about what will happen to them. Will they have to have surgery, radiation, chemotherapy? Will they die? Some patients have to face this time of illness without family or friends. When you are caring for patients with cancer, what should be your attitude? What can you say and what shouldn't you say? You are not their friend or their family. Many patients are from other cultures and may have different religions and beliefs than you. What can you do and how can you act that might be helpful and comforting and within your role as a nurse? How do these ideas about caring for patients who are critically ill and that you have probably discussed in other nursing classes relate to the medications the patient is taking and that you are administering? Discuss this as a class.

3. Do some research about the nurse practice acts in several states to learn what restrictions might apply to nurses giving antineoplastic drugs. For the states that you and your classmates check, are the restrictions the same or different?

Cardiovascular and Renal Medications

Go to http://evolve.elsevier.com/edmunds/lpn/ for additional activities and exercises.

PART I: ANTIANGINALS AND PERIPHERAL VASODILATORS

1. Vasodilators increase blood flow to the extremities by:
   1. decreasing the amount of blood carried to the heart.
   2. increasing the heart rate.
   3. relaxing the smooth muscles of the blood vessels.
   4. reducing the pressure the heart has to pump against.

2. Adverse reactions caused by nitroglycerin include: *(Select all that apply.)*
   1. flushing and headaches.
   2. postural hypotension.
   3. ringing in the ears.
   4. dizziness and fainting.

3. Drugs that interact with nitrates include: *(Select all that apply.)*
   1. alcohol.
   2. antihistamines.
   3. antidepressants.
   4. hormones.

4. Peripheral vasodilating agents are used to treat what symptoms or diseases?
   1. headaches and dizziness
   2. nocturnal leg cramps
   3. cardiac dysrhythmias
   4. Raynaud's disease

5. Vasodilator medications are used to treat pain in the legs because of their effect on:
   1. coronary arteries.
   2. peripheral venous system.
   3. peripheral arterial system.
   4. urinary system.

6. Side effects produced by peripheral vasodilating agents include:
   1. severe hypotension.
   2. anginal attacks.
   3. burning sensation under the tongue.
   4. anorexia.

7. Cardiovascular drugs affect which of the following systems? *(Select all that apply.)*
   1. urinary system
   2. cardiovascular system
   3. respiratory system
   4. endocrine system

8. Precautions needed to keep in mind when applying topical nitrates include:
   1. keep away from fire or sparks.
   2. rub the ointment into the skin.
   3. do not swim or bathe after using this route.
   4. find a hairless spot to apply the medication.

9. The cardiovascular system is made up of the:
   1. heart and blood vessels.
   2. heart, lungs, and bronchioles.
   3. heart, kidneys, and bladder.
   4. heart, brain, and spinal cord.

10. Precautions needed to keep in mind when administering nitrates include: *(Fill in the blank.)*

    1. take the patient's _____ prior to administration.

    2. instruct the patient to store medications _____.

    3. have the patient _____ prior to administration.

    4. _____ after applying topical forms of nitrates.

11. Mr. Stetson, age 69, experiences frequent attacks of angina pectoris. His blood pressure is elevated and he has glaucoma. He is also a heavy beer drinker. Mr. Stetson should:
    1. be started promptly on nitroglycerin.
    2. be started on prophylactic therapy with long-acting nitrites.
    3. not use nitroglycerin products.
    4. be instructed to quit drinking beer before treatment can begin.

12. Ms. Watson has been taking nitroglycerin patches to prevent anginal attacks. In assessing Ms. Watson before she leaves the hospital, you should instruct her on: (Select all that apply.)
    1. watching for a skin rash, itching, or irritation at the patch site.
    2. avoiding large amounts of foods that stimulate the heart and make it beat faster.
    3. burning under her tongue with use of the medication.
    4. keeping a record of every anginal attack.

13. Mr. Teldrin is recovering from an attack of angina. He will be leaving the hospital tomorrow. He has been instructed to take nitroglycerin sublingually if the anginal pain returns. You would give him which of the following additional instructions?
    1. During an attack of angina, he may repeat the dose after 5 to 10 minutes if the pain is not relieved.
    2. He can take as many tablets as necessary until relief is obtained.
    3. He should never repeat a dose, but should call the physician immediately.
    4. If the pain is not relieved 3-5 minutes after taking the first dose, he should take a second dose. A third dose may be taken in another 3-5 minutes. If the pain is not relieved, he should call an ambulance and go to the hospital.

14. If a patient does not receive relief from anginal pain after taking several nitroglycerin doses, you might suspect:
    1. tolerance to the medicine has developed.
    2. the nitroglycerin can never relieve very severe pain.
    3. a larger dose is needed.
    4. the patient may be having a myocardial infarction.

15. Discuss another possible explanation other than those in question #14 when a patient takes several nitroglycerin doses, but does not receive relief from angina pain.

16. Which of the following statements would be shared with the patient and his family before discharge?
    1. Nitroglycerin tablets are narcotics used to relieve pain.
    2. A supply of nitroglycerin should be carried with the patient in a pill container and renewed every year.
    3. Nitroglycerin tablets should be changed every 3 months because the medication loses its effectiveness.
    4. Protect the tablets from damage by using the cotton wadding in the top of the bottle to cushion them.

PART II: CARDIAC ANTIDYSRHYTHMICS

1. The usual path that an impulse from the normal pacemaker of the heart passes through is:
    1. SA node, bundle of His, Purkinje fibers, AV node, right and left bundle branches.
    2. SA node, AV node, Purkinje fibers, bundle of His, right and left bundle branches.
    3. SA node, AV node, bundle of His, right and left bundle branches, Purkinje fibers.
    4. SA node, Purkinje fibers, AV node, right and left bundle branches, bundle of His.

2. Dysrhythmias that occur and affect the heart are caused by:
    1. increased sensitivity of the cells in the pacemaker of the heart and abnormal pathways.
    2. decreased sensitivity of the cells in the pacemaker of the heart and abnormal pathways.
    3. decreased excitability of the cells in the pacemaker of the heart and abnormal pathways.
    4. lengthened depolarization of the cells in the pacemaker of the heart and abnormal pathways.

3. Class IV antidysrhythmic medications have the effect of:
   1. reducing sympathetic excitation of the heart.
   2. slowing the effective refractory period of the heart.
   3. blocking the ability of calcium to enter cells of the heart.
   4. lengthening the action potential duration.

4. Mrs. Brower comes into the hospital emergency department with a heart rate of 115 and many premature ventricular contractions (PVCs). The doctor orders quinidine for her condition. What is the action of quinidine?
   1. slowing the fast inward current of sodium
   2. blocking the ability of calcium to enter cells of the heart
   3. increasing the intake of potassium into the heart
   4. decreasing the excretion of chloride

5. The doctor orders a bolus (large IV dose) of lidocaine to be given stat to Mrs. Brower. Why would this be used along with the quinidine?
   1. Lidocaine is a class I drug and quinidine is a class II drug, which can be used together.
   2. Quinidine is a class I drug and lidocaine is a class II drug, which can be used together.
   3. Quinidine is a class III drug and lidocaine is a class II drug, which can be used together.
   4. Lidocaine is a class III drug and quinidine is a class II drug, which can be used together.

6. Mrs. St. Germaine presents with a very slow, irregular heart rate of 48, and states she has been taking propranolol (Inderal) for migraine headaches. What do you think has happened?
   1. She is having GI distress from her antidysrhythmic.
   2. She is having photosensitivity from her antidysrhythmic.
   3. She is having postural hypotension from her antidysrhythmic.
   4. She is having bradycardia from her antidysrhythmic.

7. Mrs. Dradel comes into the hospital with atrial tachycardia of 160 beats/min. Which medication might the physician order for her?
   1. adenosine (Adenocard)
   2. verapamil (Calan)
   3. dofetilide (Tikosyn)
   4. propafenone (Rythmol)

8. Important teaching points to cover for patients who will be discharged from the hospital and who are taking antidysrhythmic medications include: *(Select all that apply.)*
   1. be sure not to skip doses or double the dose.
   2. report sudden weight gain, trouble breathing, or increased coughing.
   3. use caution driving , operating heavy equipment, or doing tasks requiring alertness.
   4. it is safe to take over-the-counter medications with these drugs.

9. Toxic effects of quinidine are called *cinchonism,* and the symptoms include: *(Circle all that apply.)*

   ringing in the ears (tinnitus)

   lightheadedness and vertigo

   hypokalemia (decreased potassium)

   nausea and vomiting

10. An ECG (electrocardiogram) is often used to determine:
    1. level of potassium in the blood.
    2. heart rhythm of a patient.
    3. effect of peripheral vasodilators.
    4. force of the heartbeat.

PART III: ANTIHYPERLIPIDEMICS

1. Lipoproteins are:
   1. present in the bloodstream, circulating freely as fat globules.
   2. composed of different proportions of high-density and low-density lipids.
   3. also called *chylomicrons* and are formed during absorption of dietary fat in the intestine.
   4. synthesized by the liver and distributed by the blood to tissues throughout the body.

2. The four types of lipoprotein complexes are:
   1. chylomicrons, very low-density lipoproteins, ultralow-density lipoproteins, prothrombin protein, low-density lipoproteins.
   2. very low-density lipoproteins, ultralow-density lipoproteins, low-density lipoproteins, very high-density lipoproteins.
   3. chylomicrons, very low-density lipoproteins, low-density lipoproteins, high-density lipoproteins.
   4. cholestyramine, type 1 lipoproteins, very low-density lipoproteins, very high-density lipoproteins.

3. *Hyperlipoproteinemia* refers to:
   1. defects in lipid transport and abnormal lipoprotein pattern.
   2. activated hydroxymethylglutaryl coenzyme A.
   3. occlusive arterial disease.
   4. high levels of circulating albumin.

4. Abnormal elevations of lipids may produce:
   1. hypertension.
   2. atherosclerosis.
   3. renal disease.
   4. hepatic failure.

5. Bile acid sequestrants act by:
   1. dissolving xanthamatous lipid deposits.
   2. producing excess bile acids to be reabsorbed in the intestine.
   3. inhibiting formation of cholesterol.
   4. forming insoluble complexes with bile salts, increasing bile loss through the feces.

6. Antihyperlipidemic agents from the class of fibric acid derivatives are used to:
   1. lower triglycerides and increase HDL levels.
   2. form an insoluble compound with bile salts.
   3. increase cholesterol levels and decrease HDL levels.
   4. increase release of VLDL from the liver to plasma.

7. The drug Lovastatin is in which class of antihyperlipidemic agents?
   1. HMG-CoA reductase inhibitors
   2. fibric acid derivatives
   3. bile acid sequestrants
   4. niacin

8. Treatment for hyperlipoproteinemia includes: *(Select all that apply.)*
   1. drug therapy.
   2. diet management.
   3. exercise and weight reduction.
   4. use of anticoagulants.

9. Bile acid sequestrant preparations should be prepared by:
   1. stirring after adding the powder to a liquid.
   2. allowing the powder to dissolve in a liquid before stirring.
   3. mixing only in milk products to reduce GI upset.
   4. taking the powder in a liquid 2 hours after eating.

10. Niacin is known for causing which of the following uncomfortable side effects?
    1. constipation
    2. photophobia
    3. facial flushing
    4. tinnitus

11. Items to stress in teaching patients who are taking antihyperlipidemic medications include:
    1. patients should avoid taking any form of vitamin A supplements, because it may interfere with the drug's efficacy.
    2. use of this medication will continue until the high lipid level falls to normal.
    3. any other medication ordered by the physician should be taken at the same time as this medication.
    4. notify the doctor if you develop any bleeding or other persistent problems involved with your digestion or bowels.

PART IV: CARDIOTONIC MEDICATIONS

1. The *positive inotropic action* of digoxin refers to the ability to increase the:
   1. heart rate.
   2. force of contractions.
   3. electrical conduction.
   4. resistance.

2. Cardiotonic drugs are used to treat chronic heart failure because they help in:
   1. slowing the heart rate.
   2. increasing water loss to reduce edema.
   3. reducing the effects of other medications.
   4. speeding up contractions.

3. Symptoms of chronic heart failure include: *(Select all that apply.)*
   1. anorexia, nausea, visual changes.
   2. excessive fatigue, lethargy.
   3. rapid weight gain, shortness of breath.
   4. edema of the hands and feet.

4. Draw a circle around all the symptoms of digitalis toxicity:

   nausea   dysrhythmias   bradycardia

   visual changes   headaches   drowsiness

   productive cough   shortness of breath

   vomiting   diarrhea   extreme fatigue

5. In the event of potassium loss (such as when a patient is receiving concurrent diuretic therapy), it may be necessary to increase the dietary intake of potassium-rich foods. Put a check mark next to the foods below that are rich in potassium.

dried beans and lentils	
apples and pears	
bananas and citrus fruits	
all bran cereals	

6. The *digitalizing dose* refers to the:
   1. maintenance dose.
   2. initial loading dose.
   3. regular daily dose.
   4. dose taken digitally (by mouth instead of IM).

7. Which cardiotonic medication is used for short-term treatment of heart failure?
   1. digoxin
   2. inamrinone
   3. dobutamine
   4. milrinone

8. Mr. Doxey is receiving a digitalis preparation. You are assessing his condition to determine whether the drug therapy is working. You observe that his edema has decreased, his urinary output has increased, his weight has dropped, his pulmonary congestion has decreased, and his pulse rate is 80 beats per minute. You can infer that:
   1. chronic heart failure is still present.
   2. there is still evidence of renal impairment.
   3. digitalis therapy has been helpful.
   4. the underlying dysrhythmia is unchanged.

9. The ability of a drug to influence the velocity or speed of the electrical impulses through the heart is called:
   1. inotropic action.
   2. dromotropic action.
   3. chronotropic action.
   4. toxicity.

PART V: ANTIHYPERTENSIVES, DIURETICS, AND OTHER DRUGS AFFECTING THE URINARY TRACT

1. The organs affected in target organ damage caused by hypertension include the: *(Select all that apply.)*
   1. lungs.
   2. brain.
   3. heart.
   4. kidneys.

2. High blood pressure resulting from a known disease or other problem is called:
   1. primary hypertension.
   2. secondary hypertension.
   3. idiopathic hypertension.
   4. postural hypotension.

3. Systolic blood pressure is a reflection of:
   1. the ability of the heart to pump blood through the lungs and brain.
   2. cardiac output measured in mm Hg.
   3. the highest amount of pressure in the arterial system in mm Hg.
   4. the lowest amount of pressure in the arterial system in mm Hg.

4. Diastolic blood pressure is a reflection of:
   1. the ability of the heart to pump blood through the lungs and brain.
   2. cardiac output measured in mm Hg.
   3. the highest amount of pressure in the arterial system in mm Hg.
   4. the lowest amount of pressure in the arterial system measured in mm Hg.

5. A blood pressure of 150/94 would be classified as:
   1. normal blood pressure.
   2. prehypertension.
   3. stage 1 hypertension.
   4. stage 2 hypertension.

6. Treatment of the hypertensive patient should begin:
   1. after there is evidence of vascular disease.
   2. after the age of 50, regardless of associated disease.
   3. as soon as hypertension is detected.
   4. if the diastolic pressure is over 120 mm Hg.

7. Diuretics are used in hypertension to:
   1. promote fluid loss from the body.
   2. encourage reabsorption of sodium and chloride.
   3. flush toxic metabolites, which are causing hypertension, from the circulatory system.
   4. promote weight loss in more obese hypertensive patients.

8. Beta blockers are antihypertensive drugs that reduce blood pressure through:
   1. accelerating cardiac impulses that increase the force of cardiac contraction.
   2. limiting storage sites for norepinephrine.
   3. blocking nonselective and selective beta sites.
   4. stimulating the alpha and beta sites.

9. ACE inhibitors are used for hypertension control because they will:
   1. inhibit the enzyme that converts angiotensin I to angiotensin II.
   2. release renin into the bloodstream.
   3. vasoconstrict the adrenal cortex to increase aldosterone secretion.
   4. allow the kidneys to save sodium and water.

10. Vasodilators reduce both systolic and diastolic blood pressure through:
    1. competition with alpha-adrenergic receptor sites.
    2. increasing peripheral resistance.
    3. increased water loss.
    4. direct relaxation of vascular smooth muscle.

11. Slow channel calcium entry blocking agents work through:
    1. transferring calcium for direct relaxation of vascular smooth muscle.
    2. inhibiting the passage of extracellular calcium ions through cardiac cell membrane, producing decreased peripheral vascular resistance.
    3. increasing the permeability of the cardiac membrane to calcium.
    4. selectively increasing passage of extracellular calcium ions, which promotes diuresis.

12. The therapeutic goal of hypertension therapy is to: *(Select all that apply.)*
    1. reduce symptoms of hypertension.
    2. decrease target organ damage.
    3. reduce the blood pressure to normal or near-normal.
    4. decrease urine output.

13. What are important lifestyle changes to teach patients to try prior to drug therapy for hypertension? *(Select all that apply.)*
    1. Lose weight.
    2. Increase physical activity.
    3. Increase fat, salt, and calories in the diet.
    4. Stop smoking.
    5. Reduce alcohol intake.

14. The drug of choice to start for patients who need to add drug therapy to their plan to reduce their blood pressure is:
    1. captopril.
    2. hydrochlorothiazide.
    3. furosemide.
    4. candesartan.

15. Ways to help remember the wide variety of drugs that are used to treat hypertension involve learning common endings to each classification, which include: *(Select all that apply.)*
    1. beta blockers end in "-lol."
    2. ACE inhibitors end in "-pril."
    3. angiotensin II receptor antagonists end in "-sartan."
    4. diuretics end in "-dine."

16. Circle all the frequently associated adverse reactions of thiazide therapy:

    hyperkalemia   hypokalemia

    hyperuricemia   glucose intolerance

    impotence   cataracts   diabetes

    depression   bizarre dreams

17. Beta-adrenergic blockers are associated with adverse reactions such as: *(Select all that apply.)*
    1. bradycardia.
    2. wakefulness.
    3. fatigue.
    4. bizarre dreams.

18. Concurrent patient conditions that would limit the treatment of hypertension with beta blockers include: *(Select all that apply.)*
    1. asthma.
    2. COPD.
    3. peripheral vascular disease.
    4. sick sinus syndrome.

19. First-dose syncope is associated with which antihypertensive classification?
    1. central-acting adrenergic blockers
    2. beta blockers
    3. alpha-adrenergic blockers
    4. diuretics

20. Mr. Green has been taking furosemide 180 mg daily in divided dosages three times a day. What does he take for each dose?
    1. 100 mg per dose
    2. 80 mg per dose
    3. 60 mg per dose
    4. 40 mg per dose

21. A common effect of taking diuretics is hypokalemia. Which drug is less likely to cause this problem?
    1. chlorothiazide
    2. metolazone
    3. furosemide
    4. spironolactone

22. What condition would alpha-adrenergic receptor blockers be used for that will also affect the blood pressure?
    1. urinary frequency
    2. benign prostatic hyperplasia
    3. urinary tract analgesia
    4. urinary incontinence

23. Mr. Michaels, 76, comes in today for a routine blood pressure check. His blood pressure is 130/60 in the right arm, sitting position. He takes propranolol 20 mg twice daily. Mr. Michaels had a myocardial infarction last year, but has been without pain since that time. Today he complains of dizziness, shortness of breath, and a slow pulse. These findings may suggest that Mr. Michaels:
    1. is having another myocardial infarction.
    2. is just getting old and this is to be expected.
    3. needs to have his medication increased.
    4. is having a dosage-related reaction to propranolol.

24. Ms. Chou is to begin taking prazosin for her blood pressure, which is currently 178/96. What would you tell her about taking this medication?
    1. The drug may cause excessive drowsiness, which will pass after 2 weeks.
    2. She must take the medication while in the physician's office or hospital and remain there so her reaction to the medication can be evaluated. Some people pass out after taking the first dose of this medication.
    3. She must drink orange juice and eat potassium-rich foods with this drug.
    4. This drug may cause unusual hair growth on her body.

PART VI: FLUID AND ELECTROLYTES

1. Examples of electrolytes that circulate in the blood are: *(Select all that apply.)*
    1. albumin.
    2. potassium.
    3. platelets.
    4. phosphorus.
    5. chloride.
    6. sodium.

2. Dehydration can occur in patients because of which of the following conditions? *(Fill in the blanks.)*

    1. _____ and nausea

    2. fasting or being _____ for a long time

    3. _____ and hyperventilating

    4. _____ temperature

3. Nurses are able to prevent dehydration in patients by which of the following measures?
   1. stopping IV infusions
   2. encouraging oral fluids when appropriate
   3. drawing blood samples
   4. giving diuretics

4. Salt substitutes are used for patients who need to restrict their sodium intake. An example of these preparations is:
   1. sodium bicarbonate.
   2. Pedialyte.
   3. ammonium chloride.
   4. NoSalt.

5. Circle all the symptoms of dehydration the nurse might observe: *(Circle all that apply.)*

   dry skin   lack of sweat

   decreased urinary output   hypotension

   tachycardia   moist mucous membranes

   slow respirations   reddened face

   nervous activity of hands

Challenge Activity: Match the drug to its classification.

6. _____ digoxin
7. _____ lidocaine
8. _____ atorvastatin
9. _____ nitroglycerin
10. _____ clonidine
11. _____ captopril
12. _____ nifedipine
13. _____ hydrochlorothiazide
14. _____ phenazopyridine
15. _____ propranolol
16. _____ verapamil
17. _____ furosemide
18. _____ spironolactone

a. central adrenergic inhibitor
b. calcium channel blocker
c. potassium-sparing diuretic
d. loop diuretic
e. nitrate
f. beta blocker
g. ACE inhibitor
h. antidysrhythmic class 1B
i. urinary tract analgesic
j. thiazide diuretic
k. HMG-CoA reductase inhibitor
l. cardiotonic
m. angiotensin II receptor antagonist

PART VII: MASTERING IMPORTANT CARDIOVASCULAR WORDS AND CONCEPTS

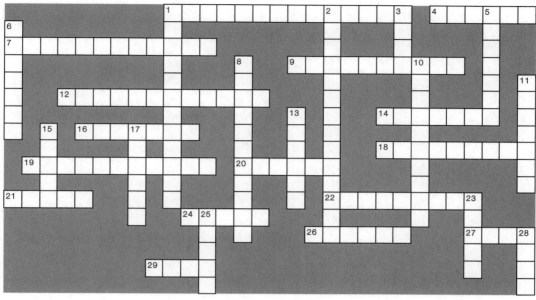

Across

1. High levels of lipoproteins in the blood.
4. Cardiac _____ is the amount of blood pumped out with each heartbeat.
7. A drug that affects the rate of the heartbeat is called a _____ drug.
9. The middle layer of the heart wall.
12. Irregular rhythm of the heart.
14. Class of drugs that lower cholesterol.
16. Statins are taken in the _____ as the body makes more cholesterol at night.
18. This is located in the SA node and sends out electrical impulses.
19. Loss of a large amount of water from the body tissues.
20. Cardiac pain.
21. Congestive _____ failure.
22. A stronger heartbeat pumps more blood and is a positive _____ action.
24. Diuretics affect _____ and electrolyte balance.
26. Angiotensin-converting _____ inhibitors.
27. A class of diuretics.
29. The initial or loading _____.

Down

1. Primary or essential _____.
2. The movement of electrolytes in and out of the cells of the heart.
3. Bile _____ sequestrants.
5. Patches of atherosclerotic tissue.
6. An extra or early heartbeat.
8. Slow heart rate, <50 beats per minute.
10. Myocardial _____ (MI).
11. Propranolol.
13. _____ bicarbonate.
15. Excess fluid that pools in dependent tissues.
17. Nicotinic acid.
23. Verapamil.
25. Many medications are cleared from the body by this organ.
28. The heart is the _____ of the circulation.

29. Mr. Yu has begun having some pain in his back while hurrying up the stairs at work. He finally went to see his physician who sent him immediately to a cardiologist. Within a few days he had a stent put into a coronary artery to reduce blockage and help decrease his risk of having a heart attack. He has always prided himself on being healthy and is very unhappy to have to change his diet, take medications, stop smoking, and lose weight. There is a lot to teach Mr. Yu. Talk with your classmates about what you believe are the most important things to teach Mr. Yu about his medications. Do you all agree? What medications are likely to be ordered? What will he need to know about them? What adverse effects might develop? Mr. Yu is from China. How would you learn if there are cultural beliefs or traditions that would influence his willingness to take medicine?

30. Sybil Wilson is 47 years old and has been diagnosed with atrial fibrillation and started on an
antidysrhythmic medication to help her heart
beat more regularly. What medication might be
ordered? What does Sybil need to know about
her medicine? Why does it matter if her heart
beats irregularly?

Central and Peripheral Nervous System Medications

chapter

13

 Go to http://evolve.elsevier.com/edmunds/lpn/ for additional activities and exercises.

Note to student: These medication sections are grouped together because many of the same drugs are found in more than one section. You will learn more about each drug and their different actions as you encounter them in different sections. It is assumed that your classes will only cover part of this chapter at one time.

These are extremely important medications to understand because many of these drugs can be toxic to the body's organ systems if they are not given correctly. A good understanding of the anatomy and physiology of the body will help in understanding the actions of these drugs.

PART I: ANTIMIGRAINE MEDICATIONS

1. The three naturally occurring catecholamines in the human body are: *(Select all that apply.)*
   1. norepinephrine.
   2. dopamine.
   3. acetylcholine.
   4. epinephrine.

2. How do antimigraine products act to reduce pain from migraine headaches?
   1. They increase vascular resistance.
   2. They increase blood pressure.
   3. They decrease the lumen of the blood vessel.
   4. They dilate the blood vessels.

3. Why are 5-HT agonists not given to patients with ischemic heart disease or other major cardiovascular problems?
   1. They can cause ringing in the ears.
   2. They can cause dizziness and vertigo.
   3. They can cause a sudden drop in blood pressure.
   4. They can cause coronary vasospasms.

4. An overdose of cholinergic drugs can cause a:
   1. release of acetylcholine.
   2. cholinergic crisis.
   3. release of epinephrine.
   4. hypertensive crisis.

5. The nurse should be alert for the following herbal medications that the patient may be taking for migraines because of potential drug interactions from prescribed medications. *(Select all that apply.)*
   1. feverfew
   2. ginkgo
   3. chamomile
   4. melatonin

6. What is often added to the antimigraine product to speed up absorption of oral and rectal preparations?
   1. aspirin
   2. acetaminophen
   3. caffeine
   4. ibuprofen

7. Abruptly stopping a migraine agent after prolonged use can result in:
   1. withdrawal symptoms.
   2. strokes.
   3. damage to the uterus.
   4. rebound headaches.

8. The patient complains of stomach upset after taking naratriptan (Amerge). What should the nurse tell her to help reduce this effect?
   1. "Don't worry, this will get better with time; it is only temporary."
   2. "I think that taking your medication with food will help relieve your discomfort."
   3. "Why don't you try lying down after taking your medicine to help relieve your symptoms?"
   4. "Pain is due to tension. You can play some soft music and turn the lights off to help you relax."

9. Which antimigraine medication is considered safe to use during pregnancy?
   1. ergotamine (Ergomar)
   2. dihydroergotamine (Migranal)
   3. Cafergot
   4. Almotriptan (Axert)

10. There are some over-the-counter medications for migraine. Why don't these medications require a prescription? Think about and explain, "If these drugs are available, why would anyone need to get a prescription for other antimigraine drugs?"

11. If someone has a really bad migraine headache and they take their medication and don't feel better, what do you think they are likely to do? Discuss with your classmates about different options for treatment. How would you teach patients to proceed?

PART II: ANTICONVULSANTS

1. Trauma, diseases, and medications might cause seizures. Put a checkmark next to all the following conditions that might cause a seizure:

pancreatitis	
head injury	
brain tumor	
dysrhythmias	
meningitis	

2. What are the four major groups of drugs used to treat seizures? *(Select all that apply.)*
   1. hydantoins
   2. antidopaminergics
   3. barbiturates
   4. succinimides
   5. benzodiazepines
   6. ergotamine derivatives

3. Barbiturates have a long duration of action and are used primarily as anticonvulsants to:
   1. increase wakefulness and alertness.
   2. reduce nerve impulses going to the brain.
   3. lower the seizure threshold.
   4. stimulate the cerebral cortex.

4. What are two most common adverse reactions to barbiturates?
   1. hyperventilation, sedation
   2. increased platelet count, grinding of teeth
   3. respiratory depression, lethargy
   4. bruising of soft tissue, myalgias

5. Put a checkmark next to the herbal products that are commonly used by patients to reduce the effects of seizures.

chamomile	
bitter melon	
black cohosh	
ginger	
ginkgo	
kava kava	
gymnema	

6. Why do older adult patients require smaller doses of barbiturates than other patients?
   1. They have a lot of other medications for other problems, which reduces the amount needed.
   2. They have built up a tolerance to the medications and need less.
   3. They metabolize the medication more slowly than younger patients.
   4. They have higher levels of albumin that bind with the medication more easily.

7. Which drug class used for seizures is both an anticonvulsant and a sedative?
   1. hydantoins
   2. benzodiazepines
   3. succinimides
   4. barbiturates

8. The nurse is reviewing an order for phenobarbital for the patient with epilepsy. Which order needs to be clarified?
   1. phenobarbital 300 mg IM three times daily
   2. phenobarbital 100 mg orally now
   3. phenobarbital 50 mg orally three times daily
   4. phenobarbital 300 mg IM now

9. Which of the following anticonvulsants is a barbiturate?
   1. ethosuximide
   2. mephobarbital
   3. phenytoin
   4. diazepam

10. Name the benzodiazepines used to treat seizures. *(Select all that apply.)*
    1. diazepam
    2. carbamazepine
    3. clonazepam
    4. clorazepate

11. Which benzodiazepine is the drug of choice in treating status epilepticus?
    1. diazepam
    2. carbamazepine
    3. clonazepam
    4. clorazepate

12. Circle the symptoms that may be caused by an overdose of benzodiazepines:

    decreased hearing   drowsiness

    confusion   increased urination

    impaired gait   grinding of teeth   weakness

13. Products that may interact with benzodiazepines include:
    1. anticoagulants, acetaminophen.
    2. anticonvulsants, alcohol, antidepressants.
    3. nonsteroidal antiinflammatory drugs.
    4. antimigraine products.

14. The patient is having daytime drowsiness. From the following list of drugs she is taking, which one is the most likely cause of this symptom?
    1. amoxicillin
    2. metoprolol
    3. phenobarbital
    4. digoxin

15. The most commonly used anticonvulsant is:
    1. phenytoin (Dilantin).
    2. phenobarbital (Luminal).
    3. diazepam (Valium).
    4. carbamazepine (Tegretol).

16. It is important to stress good oral hygiene with patients who are taking hydantoins because the medication tends to:
    1. stain the teeth.
    2. contribute to bad breath.
    3. produce gum overgrowth.
    4. make the tongue sensitive to salty foods.

17. Which class of anticonvulsants interferes with the accuracy of some laboratory tests?
    1. hydantoins
    2. benzodiazepines
    3. barbiturates
    4. succinimides

18. The nurse is reviewing an order for phenytoin (Dilantin). Which of the orders below would need to be clarified?
    1. Dilantin 100 mg orally three times daily
    2. Dilantin 100 mg orally now
    3. Dilantin 100 mg IV now
    4. Dilantin 100 mg subcutaneously three times daily

19. The nurse is reviewing the discharge instructions with the patient who is being started on phenytoin (Dilantin). What would be an important point to stress?
    1. "I know you have some concerns about taking this medication, but do not worry, it is safe."
    2. "Be careful about taking this when you are in pain, because it may worsen the pain."
    3. "You may find yourself drooling or having increased secretions that cause you to cough."
    4. "You should avoid drinking alcohol while taking this drug."

20. The nurse giving the patient phenytoin (Dilantin) notices that his eyes seem to jerk from side to side. She would know this is:
    1. common in patients taking this medication.
    2. called *presbycusis* and is an adverse effect of the medication.
    3. called *nystagmus* and is a sign of phenytoin overdosage.
    4. called *tardive dyskinesis* and will gradually disappear over time.

21. Succinimides are used primarily in the treatment of:
    1. status epilepticus.
    2. petit mal seizures.
    3. grand mal seizures.
    4. generalized seizures.

22. Adverse reactions to succinimides include:
    1. essential tremors, grand mal seizures.
    2. dizziness, night terrors, hyperactivity.
    3. sedation, weakness.
    4. hiccups, drooling.

23. Which of the following anticonvulsants are from the miscellaneous category?
    1. phenytoin (Dilantin); phensuximide
    2. phenobarbital (Luminal); diazepam (Valium)
    3. acetazolamide (Diamox); phenytoin (Dilantin)
    4. gabapentin (Neurontin); valproic acid (Depakene); carbamazepine (Tegretol)

24. The most common cause of seizures is nonadherence to the antiseizure medication regimen. Why might a person not want to take their medications? If they fall down and seriously hurt themselves during a seizure, you might think that they would be more compliant in taking their medications. This is apparently not true. Why not? How would this problem make you feel when you see the patient in the hospital many times? Talk with your classmates about this and how you might proceed.

25. What is the risk to a fetus if a mother has a seizure disorder and continues to take medication during her pregnancy?

PART III: ANTIEMETIC–ANTIVERTIGO AGENTS

1. The classifications of drugs used to treat nausea and vomiting as well as vertigo are: *(Select all that apply.)*
    1. antidopaminergics.
    2. antihistamines.
    3. 5-HT receptor antagonists.
    4. anticholinergics.

2. The nurse may need to administer medication for nausea and vomiting caused by which of the following conditions? *(Select all that apply.)*
    1. Ménière's disease
    2. radiation therapy
    3. motion sickness
    4. psoriasis

3. Which one of these medications do you recognize as an anticholinergic?
    1. metaclopramide
    2. dimenhydrinate
    3. ondansetron
    4. prochlorperazine

4. Drug products used to control vertigo include: *(Select all that apply.)*
    1. meclizine.
    2. diphenidol.
    3. dimenhydrinate.
    4. diphenhydramine.

5. The most common side effect of antihistamines is:
    1. motion sickness.
    2. hypertension.
    3. sedation.
    4. nausea.

6. What is a consequence of long-term vomiting?
    1. rebound headache
    2. dehydration
    3. allergic reactions
    4. motion sickness

7. What two herbal products are used for motion sickness? *(Select two.)*
    1. chamomile
    2. ginger
    3. ginkgo
    4. peppermint

8. What is an important consideration when giving antiemetics?
   1. When unable to take tablets orally, there are other forms of the medications.
   2. These agents are recommended for use in children.
   3. Older adults generally tolerate these medications quite well.
   4. Associated sleepiness lasts a long time so patients should take these medications only at night.

9. If medications are given to prevent motion sickness, when should patients take the medication?
   1. after they develop the motion sickness
   2. 10 minutes prior to taking any trip that will induce motion sickness
   3. 30 minutes prior to traveling
   4. 2 hours prior to taking any trip

10. Which antihistamine does not have any effect on motion sickness?
    1. meclizine
    2. diphenhydramine
    3. dimenhydrinate
    4. cyclizine

11. What form does scopolamine come in?
    1. intranasal spray
    2. oral tablet
    3. transdermal patch
    4. buccal lozenge

12. Which two classifications of antiemetic agents are most effective in treating nausea and vomiting caused by chemotherapy?
    1. antidopaminergics and antihistamines
    2. anticholinergics and antidopaminergics
    3. 5-HT receptor antagonists and antihistamines
    4. anticholinergics and 5-HT receptor antagonists

13. Are there over-the-counter products that are effective antiemetic drugs? Talk to your local pharmacist about these drugs. Which drugs do they recommend? Discuss your findings with your classmates.

PART IV: ANTIPARKINSONIAN AGENTS

1. What are the most common signs and symptoms found in patients with Parkinson's disease?
   1. shuffling gait, rigidity, rapid movements, backward-pitched gait
   2. fine muscle tremors, slow movements, rigidity, shuffling gait
   3. slow movements, rigidity, shuffling gait, backward-pitched gait
   4. rigidity, decreased intelligence, fine muscle tremors, forward-pitched gait

2. What are the two main pharmacologic actions of antiparkinsonian agents? *(Select two.)*
   1. block the uptake of acetylcholine at receptor sites
   2. block the uptake of norepinephrine at receptor sites
   3. enhance release of epinephrine in the motor centers
   4. elevate the functional levels of dopamine in motor regulatory centers

3. What is the therapeutic response desired in treatment of Parkinson's disease?
   1. maintain movement and activity and increase cognition
   2. relieve symptoms and increase cognition
   3. relieve symptoms and maintain movement and activity
   4. maintain movement and reduce double vision

4. What are the two major categories of drugs used to treat Parkinson's disease?
   1. anticholinergics and dopaminergics
   2. anticholinergics and antidopaminergics
   3. antihistamines and cholinergics
   4. anticoagulants and dopaminergics

5. Which two herbal products are used to help relieve symptoms of Parkinson's disease? *(Select all that apply.)*
   1. grape seed
   2. chamomile
   3. ginkgo
   4. ginger

6. Which antiparkinsonian agent causes tardive dyskinesia as an adverse reaction?
   1. carbidopa-levodopa (Sinemet-10/100)
   2. trihexyphenidyl (Artane)
   3. tolcapone (Tasmar)
   4. levodopa (Dopar)

7. The nurse would recognize tardive dyskinesia when she saw the patient showing:
   1. involuntary movements such as grimacing, squeezing both eyes shut.
   2. jerking of the eyes from side to side or up and down.
   3. difficulty swallowing.
   4. difficulty moving tongue to say certain words.

8. What are the early signs of toxicity in the patient taking dopaminergic agents?
   1. muscle twitching and blepharospasm (spasmodic winking)
   2. decreased sweating and muscle twitching
   3. photophobia and muscle twitching
   4. confusion and blepharospasm

9. The nurse receives an order for carbidopa-levodopa (Sinemet). Which order would need to be clarified?
   1. Sinemet 25-100 2 tablets orally every 8 hours
   2. Sinemet 25-100 1 tablet orally three times daily
   3. Sinemet 25-100 4 tablets orally every 4 hours
   4. Sinemet 25-100 1 tablet orally every 4 hours

10. Which two dopaminergic drugs are used in combination to treat Parkinson's symptoms?
    1. entacapone and bromocriptine
    2. levodopa and entacapone
    3. carbidopa and levodopa
    4. carbidopa and bromocriptine

11. Long-term use of dopaminergic and anticholinergic agents can lead to which of the following symptoms? (Select all that apply.)
    1. dystonia (impaired muscle tone)
    2. shuffling gait
    3. forward-pitched gait
    4. akinesia

12. Which antihistamine is used in the treatment of Parkinson's disease?
    1. diphenhydramine
    2. dimenhydrinate
    3. meclizine
    4. cyclizine

13. When discussing the adverse effects of antiparkinsonian agents with your patient, which of the following symptoms should be reported if they occur? (Select all that apply.)
    1. stomach upset, nausea
    2. abdominal pain and distention, constipation
    3. urinary problems
    4. intermittent winking or muscle twitching

14. It is recommended that patients who are taking antiparkinsonian agents have periodic eye exams to detect:
    1. photophobia.
    2. intermittent winking.
    3. glaucoma.
    4. exophthalmos.

15. Read about the treatment of Parkinson's disease. What is one of the biggest problems in drug treatment? Are the older drugs or the newer drugs the most effective? How many drugs control the symptoms of Parkinson's disease?

PART V: ANTIANXIETY AGENTS

1. Anxiety that requires medication treatment can create which of the following feelings? (Select all that apply.)
   1. helplessness
   2. nausea
   3. inability to concentrate
   4. irritability

2. Why should antianxiety agents be given for only a short period of time?
   1. They are addictive.
   2. They are expensive.
   3. They are only effective for a short time.
   4. They cause more anxiety if used for a long time.

3. Antianxiety agents are also used for which of the following reasons? *(Select all that apply.)*
   1. reduce hyperthyroid symptoms
   2. treatment of muscle spasm
   3. prior to electric cardioversion
   4. management of delirium tremens caused by alcohol withdrawal

4. Nurses can observe for signs of anxiety in their patients by their behavior, which may include:
   1. restlessness, muscle tremors, muscle tension.
   2. slow pulse, constricted pupils.
   3. nausea, vomiting, hair loss.
   4. lethargy, feeling of fatigue.

5. Which of the following antianxiety agents are from the classification of nonbenzodiazepines? *(Select all that apply.)*
   1. diazepam
   2. doxepin
   3. halazepam
   4. hydroxyzine

6. Benzodiazepines may cause gastrointestinal distress. What might you teach the patient about avoiding or decreasing this problem?
   1. "Take an antacid to relieve symptoms of GI distress while on your medication."
   2. "Take your medication with food to decrease GI distress."
   3. "Take half of the dose if you start to get GI distress with this medication."
   4. "Take the medication on an empty stomach to allow faster absorption."

7. The patient is receiving alprazolam (Xanax). What should the nurse tell the patient to avoid while taking this benzodiazepine?
   1. "You will need to avoid taking any herbal products, especially chamomile, as there have been reported toxicities."
   2. "You may have occasional hallucinations and feelings of confusion when you start this drug, but avoid thinking about them; these are common reactions and quickly disappear."
   3. "You should avoid smoking and drinking caffeinated beverages because they will decrease the effect of the medicine."
   4. "This drug is not habit-forming, so you can use it as long as you need it."

8. Which age groups would have the greatest potential for problems in taking benzodiazepines?
   1. 15- to 25-year-olds
   2. 25- to 35-year-olds
   3. 35- to 55-year-olds
   4. 65- to 85-year-olds

9. Which of the following functions are affected and often impaired with the use of antianxiety agents? *(Select all that apply.)*
   1. physical abilities
   2. visual and hearing functions
   3. cognitive functions
   4. mental alertness

10. Why do some people have anxiety? Often it is difficult to determine why someone is anxious. If it is a common symptom, why does it require treatment? What other things along with the medication might help reduce feelings of anxiety? Discuss this with your classmates.

PART VI: ANTIDEPRESSANT MEDICATIONS

1. What are the three major categories of medications used to treat depression? *(Select all that apply.)*
   1. 5-HT receptor agonists
   2. monoamine oxidase inhibitors (MAOIs)
   3. tricyclic antidepressants
   4. selective serotonin reuptake inhibitors (SSRIs)

2. What two antidepressants are found in the miscellaneous antidepressant category? *(Select all that apply.)*
   1. duloxetine (Cymbalta)
   2. doxepin (Sinequan)
   3. citalopram (Celexa)
   4. bupropion (Wellbutrin)

3. How are tricyclic antidepressants thought to work?
   1. They are thought to increase the reuptake of serotonin.
   2. They are thought to interfere with the release of dopamine.
   3. They are thought to interfere with the reuptake of norepinephrine and/or serotonin.
   4. They are thought to increase the release of dopamine.

4. Why have tricyclic antidepressants replaced MAOIs as the usual drugs of choice?
   1. The MAOIs are too expensive.
   2. The tricyclic antidepressants are cheaper.
   3. The MAOIs have more adverse side effects.
   4. The tricyclic antidepressants are only effective when MAOIs don't work.

5. Which two antihypertensives are not effective when used with tricyclic antidepressants?
   1. guanethidine and clonidine
   2. guanethidine and chlorothiazide
   3. clonidine and amiloride
   4. clonidine and chlorothiazide

6. What two adverse reactions are likely to occur when tricyclic antidepressants and MAOIs are used conjunctively?
   1. hypotension and hyperpyrexia
   2. hypertension and hyperpyrexia
   3. hypotension and hypothermia
   4. hypertension and hyperthermia

7. How are MAOIs thought to work?
   1. They are thought to interfere with the reuptake of serotonin.
   2. They are thought to block the inactivation of the biogenic amines.
   3. They are thought to block the release of norepinephrine.
   4. They are thought to interfere with the reactivation of biogenic amines.

8. Tricyclic antidepressants be contraindicated in which patient? *(Select all that apply.)*
   1. 45-year-old male with a history of narrow-angle glaucoma
   2. 74-year-old female with a history of renal failure
   3. 36-year-old female with a history of diabetes
   4. 62-year-old male with a history of a myocardial infarction

9. How are SSRIs thought to work?
   1. They are thought to break down serotonin as it is released.
   2. They are thought to block the inactivation of the biogenic amines.
   3. They are thought to block the release of norepinephrine.
   4. They are thought to inhibit the reuptake of serotonin.

10. Which antidepressant products have an effect on serotonin uptake but are not SSRIs? *(Select all that apply.)*
    1. bupropion (Wellbutrin)
    2. venlafaxine (Effexor)
    3. citalopram (Celexa)
    4. nefazodone (Nefazodone)

11. Which three antidepressant products are considered tetracyclic compounds? *(Select all that apply.)*
    1. venlafaxine (Effexor)
    2. maprotiline (Maprotiline)
    3. trazodone (Desyrel)
    4. mirtazapine (Remeron)

12. Which herbal product used to treat depression has the potential to interact with other antidepressants?
    1. ginger
    2. chamomile
    3. St. John's wort
    4. kava kava

13. The antidepressant amitriptyline has the common side effect of:
    1. sedation.
    2. hypotension.
    3. GI distress.
    4. photophobia.

14. Bupropion HCl (Wellbutrin) has been noted for occasionally producing what adverse reaction?
    1. tinnitus
    2. photophobia
    3. seizures
    4. anxiety

15. The SSRI citalopram (Celexa) can be effectively used for which of the following conditions? *(Select all that apply.)*
    1. depression
    2. manic-depression
    3. alcoholism
    4. panic disorder

16. For patients taking MAOIs, which of the following foods should absolutely be avoided?
    1. chicken livers, cheese, soy sauce, and decaf coffee
    2. sour cream, bananas, pickled herring, and ginger ale
    3. yogurt, raisins, fava beans, and orange juice
    4. cheese, pickled herring, avocados, and soy sauce

17. The patient complains that whenever she takes her doxepin (Sinequan) that her mouth gets very dry. To help lessen this reaction she should be told:
    1. "You should take this drug at bedtime to reduce this effect."
    2. "You could chew sugarless gum or suck on hard candy to reduce this effect."
    3. "You should drink beer with this drug to avoid that effect."
    4. "You could take this drug once a week to avoid this effect."

18. What foods cause serious reactions in patients who are taking MAO inhibitors? What kind of reactions do the patients have if they eat something they shouldn't? Make a list of those foods that are contraindicated in patients taking MAOIs. How could you teach patients about this problem so they understand the seriousness of watching their food intake? Is there anything else besides food that might be a problem for patients taking MAO inhibitors?

19. There are now many antidepressants on the market. From reading your textbook, how would you decide which one is the most helpful to patient? Why do you think so? What is your evidence? Do all antidepressants work to relieve depression? Discuss this with your classmates.

20. Some young women who are very depressed also may become pregnant. What is the risk to a fetus if the mother continues to take antidepressants while she is pregnant? Are all antidepressants a problem for a pregnant mother? What should a pregnant mother taking antidepressants be told?

PART VII: ANTIPSYCHOTIC MEDICATIONS

1. What mental illnesses are treated with antipsychotic drugs? *(Select all that apply.)*
   1. schizophrenia
   2. organic brain syndrome
   3. mania
   4. dementia

2. What is one of the major ways antipsychotic agents are thought to work?
   1. blocking the action of dopamine
   2. blocking the action of serotonin
   3. blocking the reuptake of serotonin
   4. blocking the effect of norepinephrine

3. Phenothiazines have many drug interactions. Drugs from which drug classification increase the effect of the phenothiazines?
   1. antacids
   2. beta blockers
   3. tricyclic antidepressants
   4. barbiturates

4. Antipsychotic agents produce side effects on the respiratory system, causing: *(Select all that apply.)*
   1. slow respirations.
   2. depressed cough reflex.
   3. wheezing and increased secretions.
   4. severe asthma.

5. When discontinuing phenothiazines, they should be gradually reduced over several weeks to avoid:
   1. hypotension.
   2. rebound headache.
   3. dyskinesia (involuntary muscle movements).
   4. excessive sweating.

6. Once a patient starts on a phenothiazine, how long before he or she starts getting better?
   1. The effect of the phenothiazines takes several months to start.
   2. The effect of the phenothiazines starts to work after the first dose.
   3. The effect of the phenothiazines takes several weeks to start.
   4. The effect of the phenothiazines starts to work after the fourth dose.

7. The symptoms of phenothiazine overdosage include: *(Select all that apply.)*
   1. exaggerated CNS depression.
   2. hypertension.
   3. cardiac dysrhythmias.
   4. extrapyramidal symptoms.

8. Which nonphenothiazine antipsychotic medication may cause cataracts?
   1. clozapine (Clozaril)
   2. olanzapine (Zyprexa)
   3. ziprasidone (Geodon)
   4. quetiapine (Seroquel)

9. Why should the patient taking phenothiazines avoid activities that cause excessive sweating and urination?
   1. They will make the patient perspire more than usual and get dehydrated.
   2. They will make the patient perspire less than usual.
   3. They will make the patient perspire as usual but increase the odor of the perspiration.
   4. They will make the patient perspire while at rest.

10. What are three nonphenothiazine antipsychotics? *(Select all that apply.)*
    1. clozapine (Clozaril)
    2. haloperidol (Haldol)
    3. promazine (Sparine)
    4. olanzapine (Zyprexa)

11. In order to reduce the effects of light-headedness sometimes caused by phenothiazines, the patient should:
    1. stand up as quickly as possible after lying down.
    2. move slowly from a lying position to a sitting position.
    3. drink water first before attempting to sit up.
    4. avoid lying down; sit up in a chair to sleep.

12. Some antipsychotics have occasionally been found to be used in nursing homes to inappropriately sedate patients who are troublesome to the staff. This is not a legal use of the drug. What antipsychotic medications might fall into this category? What do you think about this problem? What could/should you do about it if you see agitated patients being given inappropriate medications?

PART VIII: ANTIMANICS

1. Why is lithium unique when compared to all other psychiatric drugs?
   1. It has the most sedative actions of all the other psychiatric drugs.
   2. It alters potassium transport at the nerve endings.
   3. It has the fewest side effects and drug interactions of all the other psychiatric drugs.
   4. It is the primary drug used to treat patients in manic states.

2. Lithium overdose frequently occurs and should be suspected if the patient has: *(Select all that apply.)*
   1. restlessness.
   2. diarrhea.
   3. polyuria.
   4. muscle weakness.

3. Adverse reactions to lithium include: *(Select all that apply.)*
   1. rash.
   2. drowsiness.
   3. hypotension.
   4. weight loss.

4. When patients are in a manic state, they may exhibit symptoms that include: *(Select all that apply.)*
   1. excessive talkativeness, hyperactivity, ideas of being very powerful.
   2. slurred speech, drooping eyelids.
   3. metallic taste, red swollen tongue.
   4. severe itching, conjunctival irritation, and dry eyes.

5. An important thing for the nurse to teach the patient about lithium is:
   1. "You will need to have the level of lithium in your blood measured every 6 months."
   2. "You will need to restrict the amount of water you drink every day."
   3. "You will need to drink enough water to stay hydrated and avoid caffeine that will increase urination."
   4. "You will need to protect your skin from the sun while on lithium."

6. Which patients are not good candidates to take lithium? *(Select all that apply.)*
   1. 25-year-old female who is pregnant
   2. 10-year-old male
   3. 45-year-old female with diabetes
   4. 76-year-old male

7. The nurse is reviewing an order for lithium from the physician. Which order would need to be clarified?
   1. lithium blood levels daily
   2. lithium blood levels every 6 hours
   3. lithium blood levels before every office visit
   4. lithium blood levels every year

8. Lithium is a heavy metal and very toxic. Many children die from taking lithium that they find in their homes. How can you teach patients about this problem?

9. What do you know about bipolar depression that might lead you to believe that these patients might have a difficult time taking their lithium medications and getting the required blood work drawn? Discuss this issue with your classmates.

PART IX: SEDATIVE-HYPNOTICS

1. The term *sedative* refers to medications that cause what effect?
   1. increased wakefulness
   2. difficulty falling asleep
   3. relaxation
   4. sleep

2. The term *hypnotic* refers to medications that cause what effect?
   1. relaxation
   2. sleep
   3. increased wakefulness
   4. difficulty falling asleep

3. How could a medication used as a sedative also be a hypnotic?
   1. That is not possible, no drug can do both.
   2. The properties of the drug are related to the dosages.
   3. The main action causes sedation and the hypnotic is a side effect.
   4. This is very rare action and considered unsafe.

4. Which herbal products are used to treat insomnia? *(Select all that apply.)*
   1. valerian
   2. kava kava
   3. ginkgo
   4. chamomile

5. What is REM?
   1. REM is rapid ear movement.
   2. REM is really ear movement.
   3. REM is rapid eye movement.
   4. REM is jerking eye movement.

6. What are the classifications of insomnia? *(Select all that apply.)*
   1. intermittent insomnia
   2. terminal insomnia
   3. initial insomnia
   4. continual insomnia

7. What typical effect does the patient experience after taking sedative-hypnotics?
   1. refreshing sleep
   2. normal sleep patterns
   3. vivid and pleasant dreams
   4. increased tiredness or a "hangover"

8. The patient is complaining of not getting enough sleep and feeling anxious. She should be told:
   1. "You will need to stop taking your sleeping pill, because this is a common effect."
   2. "You are not getting enough REM sleep."
   3. "You just need to get to bed earlier."
   4. "You will have to tell your doctor, who can order a succinimide for sleep."

9. What three different groups of medications have sedative-hypnotic effects?
   1. benzodiazepines, piperidine derivatives, and hydantoins
   2. piperidine derivatives, benzodiazepines, and MAOIs
   3. benzodiazepines, tricyclic antidepressants, and phenothiazines
   4. benzodiazepines, chloral derivatives, and piperidine derivatives

10. Which classification of sedative-hypnotic medications is considered the safest group?
    1. barbiturates
    2. benzodiazepines
    3. nonbarbiturates-nonbenzodiazepines
    4. narcotics

11. Instructions for patients who are taking sedative-hypnotics should include:
    1. drink lots of water and stay hydrated when taking these drugs.
    2. increased alertness will occur immediately after taking these drugs.
    3. tolerance and dependence may develop with use of these drugs.
    4. wearing a Medic-Alert bracelet is required when taking these drugs.

12. Which medication is considered a miscellaneous sedative-hypnotic?
    1. chloral hydrate (Aquachloral)
    2. amobarbital (Amytal)
    3. zolpidem (Ambien)
    4. lorazepam (Ativan)

13. The patient says that since he left the hospital he has had a difficult time sleeping, does not feel refreshed, and has long and vivid dreams. What should the nurse tell the patient?
    1. "Don't worry; we expected that, it is not going to be a problem."
    2. "Were you taking any sleeping medications when you were in the hospital?"
    3. "Being home from the hospital always requires a period of adjustment."
    4. "Most people sleep better in the hospital than at home, so this effect will eventually improve."

14. If you were having a hard time sleeping and had access to sleeping pills from a friend, why should you or should you not take them? Is there any risk to you if you took them? Talk with your classmates about this issue.

15. Have you ever known anyone who took a sleeping pill? What was their experience? Discuss what you know about long-term use of sleeping pills with your classmates.

16. **Challenge Activity:** Read the following questions and think about the answers without sharing with your classmates. It is possible to become addicted to some types of sleeping medications. On a very personal level, do you think you have a personality that would likely lead you to become addicted to drugs? What makes you think this? As an LPN/LVN, you are going to handle medications that could cause addiction. What things are going to discourage you from ever trying these drugs? Think about this and make plans for what you will do to avoid this problem.

Medications for Pain Management

chapter

14

 Go to http://evolve.elsevier.com/edmunds/lpn/ for additional activities and exercises.

Note to student: This review chapter is designed to help you master basic content about pain medication. While drug dosages are not presented in the text, you will be asked some questions about drug dosages that you will have to look up in a drug reference book. Common drug dosages are especially important with this category of drugs to link to specific medications.

PART I: NARCOTICS

1. Narcotic agonist analgesics are used to treat which type of pain? *(Select all that apply.)*
    1. acute pain of myocardial infarction
    2. cough from the common cold
    3. pain associated with labor and delivery
    4. dyspnea related to left ventricular failure
    5. postoperative pain
    6. acute renal colic
    7. tension headache

2. What is the difference between acute pain and chronic pain?
    1. *Acute pain* refers to a prolonged onset and *chronic pain* refers to a sudden onset.
    2. Acute pain is related to prolonged drug use and chronic pain is related to intermittent drug use.
    3. Acute pain is usually related to an injury and resolves with healing; chronic pain is related to disorders which get progressively worse.
    4. *Acute pain* refers to the amount of drug needed to take effect and *chronic pain* refers to the amount of drug needed to cause adverse effects.

3. Preexisting medical problems may be adversely affected by narcotics in which of the following situations? *(Select all that apply.)*
    1. increased heart rate in patients with heart disease
    2. increased convulsions in patients with history of seizures
    3. depressed mobility in patients with arthritis
    4. depressed cough reflex in patients with lung disease

4. When the patient administers his or her own pain medication through an IV, it is referred to as:
    1. PTA medication administration.
    2. PCA medication administration.
    3. TCA medication administration.
    4. MCA medication administration.

5. One of the main side effects of narcotics is to decrease the patient's normal cough and sigh reflexes which help clear the lungs. This might lead the patient to develop:
    1. asthma.
    2. COPD.
    3. pneumonia.
    4. emphysema.

6. Narcotic agonist analgesics are metabolized by which organ?
    1. lung
    2. kidney
    3. heart
    4. liver

7. Which of the following behaviors might be considered signs of dependence on narcotics? *(Select all that apply.)*
   1. asking for pain medication every 3 to 4 hours postoperatively for 2 to 3 days
   2. requesting an increased dosage and frequency of medication administration over time
   3. receiving care for the same problem from several different physicians or agencies
   4. a history of dependence or abuse
   5. a clinical problem that produces chronic pain
   6. inability to wean from the drug

8. How are the majority of narcotics excreted from the body?
   1. through the skin in sweat
   2. through the kidneys in urine
   3. they don't leave the body; they remain in an inactive state in the tissues
   4. through the lungs during exhalation

9. How does drug tolerance differ from drug addiction?
   1. *Drug tolerance* refers to the changes in the body when a drug is stopped versus a *drug addiction* where the drug has produced psychological dependence.
   2. Drug tolerance is a psychological dependence on a drug versus drug addiction, which is a decreasing effectiveness of a drug.
   3. *Drug tolerance* refers to a decreasing effectiveness over time versus a *drug addiction* where the drug has produced a psychological dependence.
   4. *Drug tolerance* is the same as drug abuse. *Drug addiction* refers to the decreasing effectiveness of the drug over time.

10. What are signs that the patient is having pain even if he or she is unable to talk?
    1. crying, tense muscles, and sweating
    2. increased urination, fever, and hypotension
    3. regular respirations, dilated pupil reaction, and sweating
    4. slow respirations, flaccid muscles, and sweating

11. Put an X next to the most common adverse reactions and overdosage symptoms of the narcotic agonist-antagonist medications.

bradycardia	
hypotension	
constipation	
increased salivation	
enlarged pupils	
pinpoint pupils	
gasping respirations	
euphoria	

12. What are the most common narcotics used in narcotic combination products?
    1. codeine, ibuprofen, and morphine
    2. hydrocodone, codeine, and morphine
    3. codeine, acetaminophen, and aspirin
    4. codeine, oxycodone, and hydrocodone

13. What are the most frequently used nonnarcotic ingredients in narcotic analgesic combination products?
    1. aspirin, acetaminophen, and caffeine
    2. aspirin, ibuprofen, and caffeine
    3. acetaminophen, ibuprofen, and butalbital
    4. aspirin, butalbital, and caffeine

14. Mr. Sykes is recovering from surgery following a ruptured appendix. He had a severe postoperative infection with a high temperature and excessive pain. He has been receiving codeine 32 mg prn, ampicillin 500 mg four times daily, and acetaminophen 650 mg every 4 hours for the last 4 days. He is complaining of constipation. What has caused the constipation?
    1. Acetaminophen is the cause.
    2. Ampicillin is the cause.
    3. Codeine is the cause.
    4. High fever and pain are the cause.

15. What should the nurse say to the patient who is requesting that the nurse give her codeine more frequently than ordered?
    1. "I will have the physician write an order to increase the frequency for you."
    2. "Can you tell me about your pain?"
    3. "The frequency cannot be changed from what it is now."
    4. "Why don't we just back off on pain medications for now, okay?"

16. After the patient takes the first dose of a narcotic, how can the nurse help the patient prevent nausea?
    1. "You can take an antiemetic after taking the first dose to prevent nausea."
    2. "You can eat a full meal after taking the first dose to prevent nausea."
    3. "You can lie down for a short period of time after taking the first dose to prevent nausea."
    4. "You can walk around for a half an hour after taking the first dose to prevent nausea."

17. The nurse is reviewing an order for morphine for a patient who is recovering from surgery. Which order would need to be clarified with the physician?
    1. morphine 8 mg IM every 4 hours prn
    2. morphine 2 mg IV every 2 hours prn
    3. morphine 25 mg subcutaneously every 2 hours prn
    4. morphine 10 mg IM every 4 hours prn

18. You have given the patient an injection of morphine for pain. Put a check next to the symptoms below you believe are side effects of morphine.

1. hiccups	7. constipation
2. tongue swelling	8. fainting
3. nausea	9. itching
4. rapid pulse	10. skin rash
5. flushing of face	11. anorexia
6. diarrhea	12. taste of metal

19. What symptoms might you expect to see if you believed the patient had an overdose of an opioid product? Put a check next to the symptoms below you believe are correct.

1. dilated pupils	5. small constricted pupils
2. bradycardia	6. tachycardia
3. hyperventilation	7. bradypnea
4. anxiety	8. sedation

PART II: NARCOTIC AGONIST/ANTAGONIST AND NONNARCOTIC ANALGESICS

1. Which nonnarcotic central-acting analgesic is given as a continuous epidural infusion?
   1. buprenorphine (Buprenex)
   2. pentazocine (Talwin)
   3. clonidine (Duraclon)
   4. tramadol (Ultram)

2. The nurse sees an order for Oxecta, a new oxycodone product. This drug:
   1. tends to be more expensive than other products of the same classification.
   2. can be given IM, subcutaneously, or IV.
   3. contains niacin which will produce skin flushing and irritation if the normal dose is exceeded.
   4. has an onset of 15 minutes.

3. Common adverse reactions to nonnarcotic analgesics include: *(Select all that apply.)*
   1. diarrhea.
   2. disorientation.
   3. slurring of speech.
   4. postural hypotension.

4. When would the nurse need to have the nonnarcotic analgesics stopped?
   1. When the patient only has mild pain.
   2. When the drugs cause high blood pressure and rapid pulse.
   3. When the drugs cause severe insomnia.
   4. If the patient is hallucinating, confused, or loses consciousness.

5. Which narcotic agonist-antagonist analgesic medication is available in an oral form as well as injectable?
   1. pentazocine (Talwin)
   2. nalbuphine (Nubain)
   3. buprenorphine (Buprenex)
   4. butorphanol (Stadol)

6. Which two nonnarcotic analgesic products contain both aspirin and acetaminophen?
   1. Equagesic and Anacin
   2. Anacin and Vanquish
   3. Vanquish and Excedrin
   4. Excedrin and Anacin

PART III: MASTERY OF PAIN MANAGEMENT MEDICATIONS

1. Go to the Internet and search for symptoms of pain in infants and children of different ages. Discuss with your classmates specific differences in how children of different ages show pain. Do you believe that because children of different ages show pain differently, the pain should be treated differently? Where did you learn the most valuable information about this subject?

2. Newborn infant boys are often circumcised. Do they need any pain medication? Why or why not?

3. What are some hints that a patient you are interviewing might be seeking narcotics? What is "doctor shopping" and how does knowing about this condition help you in dealing with patients who might come into an office or clinic?

Antiinflammatory, Musculoskeletal, and Antiarthritis Medications

chapter

15

ⓔ Go to http://evolve.elsevier.com/edmunds/lpn/ for additional activities and exercises.

Note to student: These drugs are used in treating acute injuries and in long-term management of chronic pain. Clearly separate these conditions in your mind as you study which drugs are useful in treating musculoskeletal problems.

PART I: ANTIINFLAMMATORY ANALGESIC AGENTS

1. Salicylates have which of the following effects? *(Select all that apply.)*
   1. antiseptic
   2. analgesia
   3. antiinflammatory
   4. antipyretic

2. Aspirin has the greatest antiinflammatory effect of all salicylates. It also affects:
   1. white blood cells and factor VIII.
   2. red blood cells and factor X.
   3. platelets and factor III.
   4. lymphocytes and factor II.

3. Salicylates are most commonly used in the treatment of which of the following conditions? *(Select all that apply.)*
   1. GI bleeding
   2. pain in muscles and joints
   3. various forms of arthritis
   4. thyroid conditions

4. Which of the following are salicylates? *(Select all that apply.)*
   1. Aspergum
   2. Acephen
   3. Ascriptin
   4. Nalfon

5. Two common adverse reactions to salicylate analgesics include:
   1. tinnitus and GI bleeding.
   2. visual disturbances and metabolic alkalosis.
   3. bradycardia and anorexia.
   4. fluid retention and stupor.

6. What is the initial drug of choice in the treatment of osteoarthritis?
   1. penicillamine
   2. ibuprofen
   3. acetaminophen
   4. salicylates

7. What is one important difference between aspirin and acetaminophen?
   1. Aspirin has antiinflammatory properties and acetaminophen does not.
   2. Acetaminophen has antiinflammatory properties and aspirin does not.
   3. Aspirin has antipyretic properties and acetaminophen does not.
   4. Acetaminophen has antipyretic properties and aspirin does not.

8. Why are nonsteroidal antiinflammatory drugs (NSAIDs) contraindicated in patients who have a history of allergy to aspirin?
   1. Because aspirin can cause low toxicity in patients taking NSAIDs.
   2. Because NSAIDs are closely related to aspirin and a cross-sensitivity may develop.
   3. Because aspirin can cause worsening of joint pain in patients taking NSAIDs.
   4. Because NSAIDs can cause low toxicity in patients who react to salicylates.

9. Situations in which salicylate use might be contraindicated would include surgery, before labor, or in patients with transient ischemic attacks (TIAs) because:
    1. bleeding may be increased.
    2. weight gain may result.
    3. hypersensitivity may occur.
    4. pain may increase.

10. Reye's syndrome can occur in children who are given aspirin for symptoms of a viral illness; Reye's syndrome has the following symptoms:
    1. fever, chills, and rash
    2. diarrhea, restlessness, hyperactivity, and hypertension
    3. vomiting, lethargy, delirium, and coma
    4. joint pain and muscle weakness

11. Which vitamin is known to increase the effects of salicylates?
    1. vitamin B_1 (thiamine)
    2. vitamin K
    3. vitamin E
    4. vitamin C (ascorbic acid)

12. How does aspirin cause antiinflammatory and analgesic effects?
    1. Aspirin blocks the production of cyclooxygenase.
    2. Aspirin increases production of prostaglandins.
    3. Aspirin interferes with platelet aggregation.
    4. Aspirin inhibits the secretion of norepinephrine.

13. Which of these patients can be given salicylates?
    1. Mr. Alvarado, who has cirrhosis of the liver
    2. Mrs. Leido, who is in her second trimester of pregnancy
    3. Bobbie Feldman, age 3, who has chickenpox
    4. Sally Pederson, who has asthma

14. What will the nurse tell the patient who complains that Motrin does not work for her pain anymore?
    1. "Maybe the doctor will try another type of pain medication."
    2. "Perhaps the doctor will have to start you on aspirin instead."
    3. "Maybe the doctor will try a different NSAID, because they work slightly differently from each other."
    4. "Maybe the doctor will increase the dose until the medication does become effective."

15. COX-1, a form of cyclooxygenase, is found in which areas of the body? *(Select all that apply.)*
    1. blood vessels
    2. stomach
    3. brain
    4. kidneys

16. In diabetic patients taking salicylates, they:
    1. may give a false reading in those patients using Benedict's Clinitest for urine glucose testing.
    2. may give a false reading in those patients using a glucometer for blood glucose testing.
    3. have no effect on diabetic urine or blood tests.
    4. may cause hyperglycemia.

17. Aspirin is used for relief of pain and inflammation and is available:
    1. in special formulations for neonates.
    2. as an over-the-counter (OTC) medication.
    3. as an OTC medication and by prescription.
    4. IV for patients in severe pain.

18. Tinnitus is described as a:
    1. sharp pain in the ocular area.
    2. sensation of fullness in the ears.
    3. slight jerking movement of the eyes.
    4. ringing sensation in the ears.

19. Drugs that inhibit COX-1 and COX-2 enzymes are considered to have the property of: *(Select all that apply.)*
    1. analgesia.
    2. antiinflammation.
    3. antipyretic.
    4. antiinfection.

20. Which of the following medications are considered NSAIDs? *(Select all that apply.)*
    1. Ecotrin
    2. Clinoril
    3. Toradol
    4. Feldene

21. How is the dosage of salicylates in arthritic patients determined?
    1. Increase the dose of aspirin until the salicylate levels are at the maximum.
    2. Increase the dose of aspirin until the symptoms improve.
    3. Increase the dose of aspirin until bleeding occurs.
    4. Increase the dose of aspirin until tinnitus occurs.

22. Drug interactions between acetaminophen and hydantoin or barbiturates may increase the risk for:
    1. nephrotoxicity.
    2. hepatotoxicity.
    3. neuropathy.
    4. hyperglycemia.

23. What is the antidote for acetaminophen overdose?
    1. ketorolac
    2. activated charcoal
    3. rifampin
    4. acetylcysteine

24. For which inflammatory condition is aspirin useful in relieving symptoms? *(Select all that apply.)*
    1. acute rheumatic fever
    2. systemic lupus erythematosus
    3. myalgias (muscle pain)
    4. transient ischemic attacks

25. What are the newest recommendations about giving aspirin to a patient who may be having a heart attack?
    1. Don't give aspirin. It does not seem to work.
    2. Don't give it. It causes too many adverse reactions, such as bleeding.
    3. Give aspirin only if the patient has had a previous heart attack.
    4. Give aspirin only if the patient has not had a previous heart attack.

26. Richard Sutton has been taking NSAIDs regularly for a sports injury. He finds that the medications produce gastric irritation. The nurse might tell him that:
    1. taking the medications with food or milk might help to reduce the problems of gastric irritation.
    2. these medications should be taken on an empty stomach.
    3. gastric irritation cannot be avoided.
    4. his medication will need to be changed.

27. The patient is told to take acetaminophen (Tylenol) when he leaves the hospital. The nurse reviews the adverse reactions of this drug and tells the patient:
    1. "Tylenol is very safe because you can get it over the counter."
    2. "You need to be careful about taking this after a viral illness; it can cause Reye's syndrome."
    3. "If you develop severe pain or a high fever, contact your physician."
    4. "It should be safe for you to take as much as you want; there are very rare incidences of overdose."

28. The nurse is discussing what side effects to expect with NSAIDs. Symptoms to report to the physician would include: *(Select all that apply.)*
    1. ringing in the ears.
    2. visual disturbances.
    3. drowsiness and lightheadedness.
    4. increased alertness.

29. Periodic laboratory tests recommended for patients taking NSAIDs include: *(Select all that apply.)*
    1. hemoglobin.
    2. creatinine.
    3. red blood cell count.
    4. platelets.

PART II: SKELETAL MUSCLE RELAXANTS

1. The main actions of skeletal muscle relaxants are to:
   1. increase muscle tone and involuntary movement without loss of voluntary motor function.
   2. accelerate transmission of impulses in the motor pathway at the level of the spinal cord.
   3. interfere with the contractile mechanism of the skeletal muscle fibers (direct myotrophic blocking).
   4. contract the muscles involuntarily.

2. Skeletal muscle relaxants are used in which of the following situations? *(Select all that apply.)*
   1. relieving pain in musculoskeletal disorders involving peripheral injury and inflammation
   2. relieving pain in neurologic disorders involving peripheral injury
   3. reducing tension in joints and ligaments
   4. relief of pain in low back syndrome

3. Common adverse reactions of skeletal muscle relaxants include: *(Select all that apply.)*
   1. irritability and insomnia.
   2. polyphagia and polyuria.
   3. hypotension and syncope.
   4. flushing and tachycardia.

4. Central nervous system (CNS) depressants that are known to boost the action of skeletal muscle relaxants include: *(Select all that apply.)*
   1. hydantoins.
   2. narcotics.
   3. hypnotics.
   4. selective serotonin reuptake inhibitors (SSRIs).

5. Long-term use of skeletal muscle relaxants is not recommended because it can cause:
   1. idiosyncratic reactions.
   2. increased muscle spasms.
   3. hepatotoxicity.
   4. addiction.

6. Skeletal muscle relaxants come in which two forms?
   1. intrathecal and parenteral
   2. rectal and oral
   3. intranasal and parenteral
   4. oral and parenteral

7. Why are injectable forms of skeletal muscle relaxants viewed to be more effective than oral medications?
   1. They increase muscle tone and involuntary movements.
   2. They are better absorbed than oral medications.
   3. They induce fewer adverse reactions.
   4. They are 10 times the dose of oral medications.

8. Occasionally, an idiosyncratic (unusual) reaction may follow the first dose of a skeletal muscle relaxant. Symptoms, seen within minutes or hours of the first dose, include:
   1. severe nausea, vomiting, and weakness.
   2. temporary loss of vision, weakness, dizziness, and confusion.
   3. respiratory depression, confusion, and drowsiness.
   4. paradoxical excitation, insomnia, and tachycardia.

9. Skeletal muscle relaxants may cause which of the following? *(Select all that apply.)*
   1. hepatotoxicity
   2. nephrotoxicity
   3. ototoxicity
   4. blood dyscrasias

10. If the skeletal muscle relaxant has been given for 45 days without any signs of improvement, the physician will likely:
    1. discontinue the drug because it is not effective.
    2. increase the dosage to achieve better results.
    3. discontinue the drug due to an increased risk of hepatotoxicity.
    4. switch to another skeletal muscle relaxant because the patient may have developed tolerance to the product.

11. The patient drives a semi truck for a living. What can the nurse tell him about the cyclobenzaprine (Flexeril) that he is taking for his back spasms?
    1. "You will need to call your health care provider if you ever miss a dose."
    2. "You should avoid driving and operating heavy machinery while taking this drug."
    3. "You can take any over-the-counter medication; they will be safe to take with this drug."
    4. "You will have to quit your job because you will not be allowed to drive a truck anymore."

12. Patients should gradually reduce the dosage of skeletal muscle relaxants before stopping them to avoid what kind of symptoms?
    1. therapeutic actions
    2. withdrawal symptoms
    3. allergic symptoms
    4. adverse reactions

13. For what side effects of skeletal muscle relaxants would the patient contact a health care provider immediately? *(Select all that apply.)*
    1. dizziness or fainting
    2. shortness of breath and wheezing
    3. unusually fast heart rate
    4. relief of spasms

PART III: ANTIARTHRITIS MEDICATIONS

1. Which of the following are conventional antirheumatic drugs used in the treatment of severe rheumatoid arthritis? *(Select all that apply.)*
    1. methotrexate
    2. infliximab
    3. abatacept
    4. quinine
    5. hydroxychloroquine sulfate
    6. simethicone

2. The difference between rheumatoid arthritis and osteoarthritis is that rheumatoid arthritis is a:
    1. more local process and osteoarthritis is a systemic disease.
    2. systemic disease and osteoarthritis is a more local process.
    3. result of overuse and osteoarthritis is an autoimmune response.
    4. result of overuse.

3. Patients who suffer from arthritis find:
    1. great difficulty getting good relief from antiarthritis drugs.
    2. it helpful to use acupuncture instead of drugs.
    3. using antiarthritis drugs works best for symptom relief.
    4. the drugs prescribed help with the swelling, but not the pain.

4. Which herbal products are popular to use in the treatment of osteoarthritis? *(Select all that apply.)*
    1. chondroitin
    2. glucosamine
    3. bromelain
    4. ginger

5. What are the first-line drugs used for the treatment of arthritis?
    1. salicylates and NSAIDs
    2. DMARDs and SSRIs
    3. beta-blockers and antidysrhythmics
    4. narcotics and antiemetics

6. Which antiarthritis drug has the FDA warning label on it that alerts health care providers not to give to pregnant women?
    1. infliximab
    2. anakinra
    3. methotrexate
    4. acetaminophen

7. This arthritis medication is toxic to the bone marrow and used for patients who are unresponsive to other treatments.
    1. anakinra
    2. acetaminophen
    3. hydroxychloroquine sulfate
    4. methotrexate

8. Which antiarthritis drug is also considered an antimalarial drug?
    1. methotrexate
    2. sulfasalazine
    3. quinine
    4. hydroxychloroquine sulfate

9. What is a potential irreversible side effect from taking hydroxychloroquine sulfate?
    1. nephropathy
    2. retinopathy
    3. ototoxicity
    4. anaphylactic shock

PART IV: ANTIGOUT AGENTS

1. A uricosuric agent is a drug that:
   1. increases excretion of uric acid.
   2. reduces the inflammation caused by gout.
   3. increases uric acid levels in the blood.
   4. increases tubular reabsorption of urate.

2. What two mechanisms produce high uric acid levels in the body?
   1. underproduction and overexcretion
   2. overproduction and overexertion
   3. overproduction and underexcretion
   4. underproduction and underexcretion

3. What other medications in addition to urico-surics are used in treating patients with acute high uric acid levels?
   1. antiinflammatories and diuretics
   2. antiinflammatories and analgesics
   3. antiinfectives and diuretics
   4. antidepressants and muscle relaxants

4. Probenecid has another action not related to gout. It acts to:
   1. increase levels of penicillin.
   2. increase levels of aspirin.
   3. decrease levels of penicillin.
   4. decrease levels of aspirin.

5. Which antigout medication is often not started unless the patient does not respond to all other drugs?
   1. colchicine
   2. sulfinpyrazone
   3. allopurinol
   4. probenecid

6. Which antigout medication inhibits the production of uric acid?
   1. colchicine
   2. probenecid
   3. allopurinol
   4. calamine

7. Gout caused by uric acid forming crystals in the kidneys and joints presents with what symptoms? *(Select all that apply.)*
   1. soft glow emanating from the area of crystals
   2. severe pain in the area of crystals
   3. warmth and increased heat in the area of crystals
   4. inflammation in the area of the crystals

8. What is traditionally the major drug used for treatment of gouty attacks?
   1. allopurinol
   2. penicillin
   3. colchicine
   4. probenecid

9. Uricosuric agents are started:
   1. usually after more than one acute attack.
   2. after the first attack.
   3. only after other agents have been tried.
   4. after kidney stones are documented by flat plate x-ray.

10. The joint in which gouty attacks occur in at least 50% of the cases is the:
   1. phalangeal.
   2. metacarpal.
   3. metatarsal.
   4. podagra.

PART V: MASTERING ANTIINFLAMMATORY, MUSCULOSKELETAL, AND ANTIARTHRITIS MEDICATIONS

1. Talk with your classmates about any musculoskeletal problems someone they have known has had in the past. When did the pain bother them the most? What did they do for it? What was the most helpful thing for them to do to cope with the pain?

2. Go to the Internet and find at least two different descriptions of pain people have with gout. What is similar and what is different about the descriptions?

3. This textbook does not list the dosages of medications even though that is one of the most important things to know. Use a drug reference text such as the *Physician's Drug Reference* or an Internet database to look up the dosages for acetaminophen. What did you learn? Can you understand why the dosages might not be listed for medications in this book? Where would you go to get the best information about dosages for different drugs?

Student Name_____ Date_____

Gastrointestinal Medications

chapter 16

 Go to http://evolve.elsevier.com/edmunds/lpn/ for additional activities and exercises.

PART I: ANTACIDS, H₂-RECEPTOR ANTAGONISTS, PROTON PUMP INHIBITORS

1. How may antacids cause hypermagnesemia?
   1. They contain magnesium.
   2. They prevent the body from using magnesium.
   3. They stimulate the production of increased amounts of magnesium.
   4. They reduce the body's need for magnesium.

2. If a patient is taking an anticoagulant, which H₂ histamine blocker is most likely to interfere with the anticoagulant?
   1. nizatidine (Axid)
   2. cimetidine (Tagamet)
   3. famotidine (Pepcid)
   4. ranitidine (Zantac)

3. The patient who is starting on a proton pump inhibitor (Protonix) asks when the best time would be for her to take the medication. Your response will be, "You should take your Protonix:
   1. at bedtime."
   2. with your meals."
   3. after meals."
   4. before meals."

4. Which drug classification is considered first-line therapy in the treatment of peptic ulcer disease?
   1. histamine H₂ blockers
   2. antacids
   3. proton pump inhibitors
   4. histamine H₂ agonists

5. For which of the following gastric conditions are antacids used as treatment? (*Select all that apply.*)
   1. gastritis
   2. peptic esophagitis
   3. esophageal reflux
   4. stomach cancer

6. Match the GI drug with its action by putting an "X" in the column corresponding to the correct response.

Drug	Decrease gastric acid secretion	Increase tone of sphincter	Promote healing of ulcers	Buffer gastric acid	Block histamine
magaldrate (Riopan)					
ranitidine (Zantac)					
pantoprazole (Protonix)					
aluminum carbonate (Basaljel)					
famotidine (Pepcid)					
omeprazole (Prilosec)					

7. Why do you think that it might be important for you as a nurse to know the answers to the questions in #6? In what job would knowing this information be especially important?

PART II: ANTICHOLINERGICS, ANTISPASMODICS, ANTIDIARRHEALS

1. Which drug classifications are used to treat both diarrhea and increased bowel motility? *(Select all that apply.)*
   1. antitussives
   2. antispasmodics
   3. anticholinergics
   4. antidiarrheals
   5. antiinfectives

2. The primary use of anticholinergic-antispasmodic agents is to treat: *(Select all that apply.)*
   1. irritable colon.
   2. diarrhea.
   3. peptic ulcer.
   4. constipation

3. The patient has been started on antidiarrheals. The primary action of antidiarrheals is to:
   1. reduce the irritability of the bowel and reduce the motility of the GI tract.
   2. increase the amount of water in the stool and increase peristalsis.
   3. reduce the amount of water in the stool and decrease peristalsis.
   4. neutralize gastric acid and increase peristalsis.

4. Mr. Frank, age 84, comes in to the clinic with mild abdominal discomfort, increased flatus, and watery stools. His history includes mild prostatic hypertrophy. Which of the following medications could be used to treat his diarrhea?
   1. bisacodyl (Dulcolax)
   2. metoclopramide (Reglan)
   3. mepenzolate (Cantil)
   4. sulfasalazine (Azulfidine)

5. Which kind of drugs would be contraindicated in the treatment of Mr. Frank because it can cause urinary retention?
   1. antidiarrheals
   2. anticholinergics
   3. antispasmodics
   4. cathartics

6. You are reviewing an order for metoclopramide (Reglan) for your patient. When would you be likely to give this medicine?
   1. every 4 hours
   2. before meals
   3. before meals and at bedtime
   4. bedtime

7. Which antidiarrheal is not available over the counter?
   1. bismuth subsalicylate (Bismatrol)
   2. diphenoxylate and atropine sulfate (Lomotil)
   3. loperamide (Imodium)
   4. kaolin and pectin (Kaopectate)

8. Antidiarrheal medications are important to control diarrhea which, if prolonged, can lead to:
   1. electrolyte imbalance and dehydration.
   2. urinary retention.
   3. increased urination.
   4. overhydration.

9. Anticholinergic medications reduce GI tract discomfort by the following action. *(Select all that apply.)*
   1. increase intestinal motility
   2. decrease intestinal motility
   3. increase acid production
   4. slow gastric emptying time

10. Common adverse reactions to anticholinergic therapy include:
    1. constricted pupils, soreness of tongue and corners of mouth.
    2. dysarthria, muscle weakness.
    3. slow, weak pulse.
    4. dysphagia; rapid, weak pulse; and dilated pupils.

PART III: LAXATIVES

1. Which major groups of laxatives are useful for patients who should not strain while having a bowel movement?
   1. bulk-forming laxatives and stimulant laxatives
   2. lubricant laxatives and fecal softeners
   3. lubricant laxatives and stimulant laxatives
   4. fecal softeners and saline laxatives

2. What conditions would be considered a contraindication for giving laxatives?
   1. anorexia, dysphagia
   2. benign prostatic hypertrophy
   3. constipation, fecal impaction, intestinal ulcerations
   4. hiatal hernia, esophageal reflux

3. Why might laxatives that contain sodium be contraindicated in a patient with chronic heart failure?
   1. They may increase irritable bowel syndrome symptoms.
   2. They can lead to an increase in cardiac symptoms.
   3. They may lead to the overuse of the laxatives.
   4. They may cause an increase in gastric distress.

4. What are the most common adverse reactions that can occur with all laxatives?
   1. urticaria and nausea
   2. diarrhea and vomiting
   3. obstructions and nausea
   4. abdominal cramping and diarrhea

5. Emulsoil is an example of what type of laxative?
   1. fecal softener
   2. bulk-forming
   3. lubricant
   4. hyperosmolar

6. The patient is taking senna for constipation resulting from taking narcotics. What should the nurse teach him about this drug?
   1. "You need to drink a full glass of water with this medication."
   2. "You need to take your antacids 1 hour prior to taking this medication."
   3. "You need to be aware that your stool may change color to yellow."
   4. "You need to take this medication with fruit juice to disguise the taste."

7. Which drug is one of the bulk-forming laxatives?
   1. docusate (Colace)
   2. bisacodyl (Dulcolax)
   3. senna (Senokot)
   4. methylcellulose (Citrucel)

8. Which laxative may take the longest to work?
   1. psyllium seed (Metamucil)
   2. docusate (Colace)
   3. senna (Senokot)
   4. bisacodyl (Dulcolax)

PART IV: MISCELLANEOUS GASTROINTESTINAL DRUGS

1. Antiflatulents are used to treat which of the following conditions?
   1. stomach cancer
   2. excess gas formation and bloating
   3. constipation
   4. diarrhea

2. Which of the following GI medications is used to treat gallstones?
   1. ursodiol (Actigall)
   2. disulfiram (Antabuse)
   3. apomorphine (Apokyn)
   4. pancreatin (Creon)

3. What are digestive enzymes used for?
   1. increased flatulence
   2. to induce vomiting
   3. to reduce diarrhea and flatulence
   4. replacement therapy

4. How often should pancreatic enzymes be given?
   1. 2 hours after eating
   2. as needed when indigestion occurs
   3. with meals and snacks
   4. only at bedtime

5. When a patient has disulfiram ordered, the condition he is suffering from is:
   1. ulcerative colitis.
   2. pancreatitis.
   3. cystic fibrosis.
   4. alcoholism.

6. This herbal product is used for treatment of heartburn/indigestion.
   1. grapefruit seed extract
   2. milk thistle
   3. ginger
   4. evening primrose

PART V: MASTERING GASTROINTESTINAL MEDICATIONS

1. There is a lot in the medical literature about young women who binge and purge and have other types of eating disorders. Go to the Internet to learn if men have any similar types of problems. If so, what symptoms would you look for? What things in the patient's history or physical exam might make you suspicious that the patient (male or female) might have an eating disorder?

2. Bowel habits are very personal. What is normal for one individual might be seen as abnormal in another. You might feel uncomfortable asking questions about bowel habits. Talk with your classmates about different ways to ask questions about bowel habits, what words to use, how to make patients feel comfortable sharing this information, and what words might be appropriate for different age groups. What can you say when you believe that the bowel patterns really are not healthy?

Hematologic Products

Go to http://evolve.elsevier.com/edmunds/lpn/ for additional activities and exercises.

PART I: ANTICOAGULANTS

1. The nurse explains to the patient that a clot formed from fibrin, platelets, and cholesterol that either attaches to the inner wall of a blood vessel or occupies the entire lumen (or inside) of a vessel is called:
   1. a thrombus.
   2. fibrinogen.
   3. thromboplastin.
   4. an embolism.

2. The patient understands that a blood clot that develops in the lower extremities and can travel through the circulation is called:
   1. thromboplastin.
   2. coagulation factors II, VII, and X.
   3. a thromboembolism.
   4. a thrombus.

3. Heparin's mechanism of action includes:
   1. interfering with the metabolic functions of vitamin K.
   2. interfering with the formation of thrombin.
   3. dissolving existing blood clots and preventing the extension of thrombi.
   4. increasing the formation of fibrin by acting on fibrinogen to trap red blood cells.

4. In order to maintain a constant level of heparin in the blood, it should be administered in which of the following ways?
   1. orally
   2. subcutaneously
   3. intermittent IV infusion
   4. continuous IV infusion

5. The nurse is reviewing an order for heparin. Which order would you need to clarify prior to giving?
   1. heparin 5000 units subcutaneously every 12 hours
   2. heparin 2000 units bolus IV now
   3. heparin 2500 units orally now
   4. heparin 1200 units/hr IV

6. The most commonly used laboratory test to monitor the effectiveness of heparin is:
   1. prothrombin time.
   2. Lee-White clotting time.
   3. partial thrombin time.
   4. activated partial thromboplastin time.

7. Oral coumarin therapy is prescribed when:
   1. the patient is not responsive to heparin therapy.
   2. the blood clots need to be dissolved.
   3. long-term anticoagulant therapy is warranted.
   4. an immediate effect of an anticoagulant is needed.

8. Coumarin acts by:
   1. interfering with the metabolic function of vitamin K.
   2. interfering with the formation of thrombin.
   3. interfering with the formation of thrombin and limiting platelet aggregation.
   4. increasing the effectiveness of heparin sodium.

9. The laboratory test that monitors the effectiveness of Coumadin is: (Select all that apply.)
   1. Lee-White clotting time.
   2. International Normalized Ratio (INR).
   3. partial thrombin time.
   4. prothrombin time.

10. A 72-year-old nursing home resident is suffering from Alzheimer's disease, and shows marked confusion. He develops acute thrombophlebitis in his left leg. There are no signs of abnormal bleeding or other conditions that would prevent anticoagulant therapy. Read about this condition and decide which medication below is most likely to be started first.
    1. heparin subcutaneously
    2. low-molecular–weight heparin
    3. Coumadin
    4. protamine sulfate

11. Ms. Watson has an acute peptic ulcer and chronic recurrent arterial occlusion in her leg. To help prevent arterial occlusion, she should:
    1. be started on coumarin therapy, but not heparin.
    2. be started on heparin therapy, but not Coumadin.
    3. not be started on either heparin or Coumadin.
    4. be started on protamine sulfate.

12. A sign of internal bleeding that may occur with anticoagulants is: *(Select all that apply.)*
    1. vomiting "coffee-ground" emesis.
    2. black, tarry stools.
    3. euphoria or confusion.
    4. abdominal swelling.

13. Which preparation is a low-molecular–weight heparin?
    1. dalteparin sodium (Fragmin)
    2. alteplase (Activase)
    3. abciximab (Reo-Pro)
    4. clopidogrel (Plavix)

14. An early sign of overdosage of anticoagulants is:
    1. hypothermia.
    2. GI upset.
    3. nosebleed.
    4. constipation.

15. What is one of the important uses of low-molecular–weight heparins?
    1. increase the formation of fibrin clots
    2. prevent atrial fibrillation
    3. dissolve existing clots
    4. prevent deep vein thrombosis after surgery

16. Why would a patient receive heparin instead of Coumadin?
    1. To convert an embolism to a thrombus.
    2. To start on long-term anticoagulation therapy.
    3. An immediate effect of an anticoagulant is needed.
    4. A blood clot needs to be dissolved.

17. When is protamine sulfate used? *(Select all that apply.)*
    1. When the patient's PT/INR is too low.
    2. In cases of heparin overdose.
    3. When the patient's aPTT is too low.
    4. When the effects of heparin need to be reversed in cases of severe bleeding.

18. What are common signs of anticoagulant overdosage? *(Select all that apply.)*
    1. nosebleeds
    2. coughing up blood
    3. bleeding gums
    4. food craving for green leafy vegetables

19. What effect do antihistamines, digitalis, and nicotine have on heparin in the hospitalized patient?
    1. They decrease the adverse reactions that can occur with heparin.
    2. They increase the anticoagulant effect of heparin.
    3. They increase the time it takes for protamine to take effect.
    4. They decrease the anticoagulant effect of heparin.

20. How is the dosage of anticoagulant medication determined? *(Select all that apply.)*
    1. Heparin infusions are weight-based for more accurate dosing.
    2. Coumadin requires repeated blood draws to determine the PT and/or INR.
    3. Heparin infusions are based on the protime of the patient.
    4. Coumadin dosages are weight-based.

PART II: THROMBOLYTIC AND ANTIPLATELET AGENTS

1. In which conditions would thrombolytic products be used? *(Select all that apply.)*
   1. chronic venous occlusions
   2. clots that are blocking coronary arteries
   3. acute arterial occlusions
   4. clots that are causing acute pulmonary emboli

2. Which of the following thrombolytic agents are used to clear IV catheters that are obstructed with a clot?
   1. alteplase (Activase)
   2. reteplase (Retavase)
   3. antithrombin III (ThrombateIII)
   4. streptokinase (Streptase)

3. In addition to bleeding, what other adverse reactions may you see in your patients who have had thrombolytic agents given to break up clots? *(Select all that apply.)*
   1. hyperthermia
   2. hypotension
   3. tinnitus
   4. dysrhythmias

4. When Mr. Adams visits his doctor for a routine examination and ECG, it is discovered that he has had a silent myocardial infarction (MI) sometime within the last few months. He asks the nurse if he will be given any "clot busters." The nurse's response may be:
   1. "I will ask the doctor that question; maybe we should give you some."
   2. "Those medications are too expensive; I think the doctor wants to save you money."
   3. "We give those clot-buster medications within 6 hours of having a heart attack, and you had your heart attack a while ago."
   4. "Why don't I check it out? As long as you are not bleeding now, we could do that for you."

5. Which one of the following miscellaneous products is used to treat sickle cell anemia?
   1. antihemophilic factor (Hemofil M/E)
   2. hydroxyurea (Droxia)
   3. tirofiban (Aggrastat)
   4. eptifibatide (Integrilin)

6. Mrs. Winters is rushed to the hospital with signs of an acute ischemic stroke. She is given a thrombolytic agent by the physician as soon as she arrives in the emergency department. The nurse is carefully monitoring her for signs of bleeding. Which sign of bleeding indicates overdosage? *(Select all that apply.)*
   1. bleeding at the infusion site
   2. hematemesis
   3. hematuria
   4. abdominal tension

7. How do thrombolytics and antiplatelet agents differ?
   1. Thrombolytics cause the breakdown of fibrin clots, but antiplatelets prevent the formation of a clot.
   2. Thrombolytics prevent the breakdown of fibrin clots, but antiplatelets cause the formation of a clot.
   3. Thrombolytics inhibit the breakdown of fibrin clots, but antiplatelets interfere with the formation of a clot.
   4. Thrombolytics limit the breakdown of fibrin clots, but antiplatelets inhibit the formation of a clot.

8. If a patient with a previous MI is suspected of having another MI, what medication can be administered immediately?
   1. clopidogrel 75 mg orally
   2. aspirin 300 or 325 mg orally
   3. alteplase 10 mg IV
   4. heparin 5000 unit IV bolus

9. The nurse is teaching the patient who will go home on Coumadin dietary considerations concerning vitamin K. What should the patient be told?
   1. "You need to be taking a vitamin supplement that has vitamin K to increase the effectiveness of this drug."
   2. "You can eat green leafy vegetables like spinach and broccoli; it is the sudden increase in the diet that will affect your medications, as well as taking vitamin supplements that have vitamin K in them."
   3. "Your diet is not important, you can eat anything you like. Just be careful with taking vitamin supplements."
   4. "You need to be aware that eating green leafy vegetables can make the side effects of this drug worse."

10. When is a thrombolytic agent used in an acute MI?
    1. when the patient is hemodynamically stable
    2. when the patient has been experiencing symptoms of severe angina for less than 12 hours and has ST-segment elevations or new left bundle branch block
    3. If symptoms have lasted less than 6 hours
    4. These medications are contraindicated if the patient is having an MI.

11. What is the dose of aspirin that is given on the way to the hospital for a patient who has no GI problems, has had an MI, and is suspected of having another MI?
    1. 250 mg
    2. 81 mg
    3. 160 to 325 mg
    4. 600 mg

PART III: MASTERING HEMOTOLOGIC PRODUCTS

1. When you practice drawing up heparin in the syringe, you notice that the amount of heparin given is a very small dose. Because it is a small dose, what might be the response if you made a mistake and gave more heparin than ordered? What might happen if you didn't give enough heparin? What steps do you take to make sure you always give the right dose?

2. Why do you not pull back on the plunger of the syringe when giving heparin? Look on the Internet to see if you can find out any other information that might be important to know in drawing up and injecting heparin. Discuss what you have found with your classmates.

3. When patients take anticoagulants, they are told to watch for signs of bleeding. Go to a textbook or the Internet and find out where patients might be bleeding if their anticoagulant dose is too high. If you are worried that the patient might be bleeding, how could you find out? Discuss this problem with your classmates.

4. The patient was told that he had a narrowing of his coronary artery, and the surgeon put in a stent (a small mesh tube used to widen narrow coronary arteries). The patient was told by the nurse that he must take clopidogrel (Plavix) every single day without fail. He must never stop taking it unless the cardiologist tells him he can stop. Why is clopidogrel ordered? Is it correct that he must never stop taking it? Why or why not? What information do you think is important to teach the patient about this drug? Discuss this with your classmates.

Hormones and Steroids

chapter
18

Go to http://evolve.elsevier.com/edmunds/lpn/ for additional activities and exercises.

PART I: INSULIN AND ORAL ANTIDIABETIC AGENTS

1. Insulin is what type of chemical?
   1. polypeptide
   2. hormone
   3. steroid
   4. neurotransmitter

2. How does insulin help lower the blood sugar?
   1. It decreases the production of sugar.
   2. It carries the sugar out of the body.
   3. It allows movement of sugar into the cells.
   4. It acts as a feedback messenger to convert protein into energy.

3. Insulin is necessary for the metabolism and use of glucose in the body and is produced where?
   1. in the lungs by the alveoli
   2. in the kidneys at the loop of Henle
   3. in the liver by the hepatocytes
   4. in the pancreas by the beta cells

4. If the patient gives frequent injections of insulin into the same site, what may be the result?
   1. polyuria
   2. lipodystrophy
   3. Somogyi effect
   4. systemic acidosis

5. If a type 1 diabetic patient begins taking oral contraceptives, is there a change in the need for insulin?
   1. No, there is no change in the need for insulin.
   2. Yes, there is often an increased need for insulin.
   3. Yes, there is a decreased need for insulin.
   4. No, there is an increased production of insulin.

6. Mrs. Halifax is a brittle diabetic (one whose blood sugar responds with wide variations in response to insulin). The nurse must watch her carefully for symptoms of hypoglycemia after giving her an insulin injection. What are the signs and symptoms of hypoglycemia? *(Select all that apply.)*
   1. cold, clammy skin
   2. hunger
   3. diaphoresis
   4. lethargy
   5. increased urination

7. Mr. Primrose often does not take his insulin at the correct time, and he skips doses when he gets busy. He is at risk for hyperglycemia. What are the signs and symptoms of hyperglycemia? *(Select all that apply.)*
   1. polymyalgia
   2. polyuria
   3. polyphagia
   4. polydipsia

8. The American Diabetes Association recommends treatment that focuses on normalizing diabetic glucose levels. What is one way that this can be accomplished?
   1. switching all diabetics to insulin
   2. open-loop insulin pumps
   3. a routine of one injection per day
   4. avoiding insulin but exercising hard

9. One function of insulin is to allow glucose into the cells. What are some other important functions? *(Select all that apply.)*
   1. inhibit lipoprotein lipase
   2. convert complex compounds to simple substances
   3. prevent release of fatty acids
   4. promote glucose transport and storage

10. In counseling Mrs. Wilson, a newly diagnosed diabetic, the nurse discovers that she has been administering regular insulin deep IM just before meals. She seems to have confidence in giving the injection and can draw up and read the dosage properly. What suggestions would you give her?
    1. "You are having some problems. I will ask the doctor to change you to an oral agent, okay?"
    2. "You are doing a nice job with drawing up and reading your insulin dose. I see you are doing everything well."
    3. "You need to be giving your injection subcutaneously, not in your muscle. Let's review that technique."
    4. "You should start to inject your medication after meals because that will give you better coverage of the food you eat."

11. The oral incretion agents help patients control their blood sugar and also have the effect of: *(Select all that apply.)*
    1. stimulating glucagon secretion.
    2. protecting the beta cells from cytokine injury.
    3. decreasing gastric emptying time.
    4. suppressing the appetite and inducing satiety.

12. The doctor decides to order a combination of regular and NPH insulin for Mrs. Wilson. It is important to tell Mrs. Wilson to:
    1. shake the insulin vial well before withdrawing the medication to make certain all chemicals are dissolved.
    2. draw up the regular insulin before drawing up the NPH insulin in the same syringe.
    3. use a different syringe for each injection.
    4. keep the insulin refrigerated until ready to use.

13. The patient asks the nurse why she has to take both insulin and an oral hypoglycemic agent to control her blood sugars. The best response for the nurse is:
    1. "You are a very brittle diabetic, and we need to use both forms of control to get your sugar level normal."
    2. "The oral agent and the insulin work differently to help control your blood sugar; it is to help you gain better control."
    3. "The doctor prescribed it this way. Maybe we'd better ask her to explain it."
    4. "You can alternate taking the insulin one day and the oral agent the next to control your sugars."

14. Mrs. Wilson is instructed to test her sugar level at home to determine how much insulin she is to take. She will do this by using a glucometer to test:
    1. blood glucose levels.
    2. urine sugar levels.
    3. both the blood and urine levels.
    4. the insulin levels.

15. Somogyi effect occurs when the patient's:
    1. blood sugar drops after being hyperglycemic.
    2. level of insulin is decreased with the use of oral agents.
    3. level of insulin is increased with the use of oral agents.
    4. blood sugar rebounds higher after being hypoglycemic.

16. The most common adverse reactions with oral hypoglycemic agents are: *(Select all that apply.)*
    1. GI symptoms.
    2. allergic reactions
    3. high blood pressure.
    4. hypoglycemia.

17. Benny Parks is a 45-year-old homeless alcoholic. He is well known to the local hospital because of his diabetes. Because he was unable to take insulin while living on the streets, the doctor started him on a sulfonylurea. What would the nurse be most concerned about?
    1. The medication requires that it be taken with food, and Benny may not be eating.
    2. The patient must eat three regular meals a day while taking this medication.
    3. A disulfiram-like reaction may result in some patients if the patient takes sulfonylureas and drinks alcohol.
    4. He will need to use a glucometer to test his blood sugar, and he has nowhere to set up the machine.

18. Miss Eldredge is a 64-year-old retired schoolteacher. She has recently been diagnosed with type 2 diabetes. The most important thing to tell her is that:
    1. a patient who has type 2 diabetes will never have to take insulin.
    2. she can avoid taking any medication if she will eliminate all carbohydrates from her diet.
    3. medication and diet are both important parts of the treatment plan.
    4. there is no cure and she will only get worse as time goes on.

19. Which of the oral hypoglycemic agents below is in the class of biguanides?
    1. acarbose
    2. metformin
    3. repaglinide
    4. glipizide

20. Which blood test is used to assess the patient's ability to control her blood sugar in recent months?
    1. hemoglobin A_{1c}
    2. hematocrit
    3. liver enzymes
    4. complete blood count

PART II: DRUGS ACTING ON THE UTERUS

1. Mrs. Ott comes into the hospital in labor. Her baby is not due for 6 more weeks. The doctor will most likely order:
    1. an abortifacient.
    2. a uterine relaxant.
    3. a muscle relaxant.
    4. an oxytocic or ergot preparation.

2. Following delivery of the baby and placenta, the uterus must clamp down to control bleeding. A medication that might help limit uterine bleeding would be:
    1. an abortifacient.
    2. a uterine relaxant.
    3. a muscle relaxant.
    4. an oxytocic.

3. Medications given to help stimulate milk to flow include:
    1. oxytocics.
    2. muscle relaxants.
    3. tranquilizers.
    4. diuretics.

4. A medication used to expel the fetus from the pregnant uterus, used early in pregnancy, is called:
    1. an abortifacient.
    2. a uterine relaxant.
    3. a muscle relaxant.
    4. an oxytocic.

PART III: PITUITARY AND ADRENOCORTICAL HORMONES

1. Pituitary hormones are important for which of the following body functions? *(Select all that apply.)*
    1. stimulate the production of insulin
    2. electrolyte balance
    3. metabolism
    4. create the reproductive cycle

2. The adrenal cortex produces which of the following substances? *(Select all that apply.)*
    1. glucocorticoids
    2. estrogens
    3. somatotropin
    4. mineralocorticoids

3. One of the anterior pituitary hormones, adrenocorticotropic hormone (ACTH), stimulates the adrenal cortex to secrete: *(Select all that apply.)*
    1. corticosterone.
    2. oxytocin.
    3. aldosterone.
    4. cortisol.

4. Corticosteroids are commonly given for the following reasons. (*Select all that apply.*)
   1. increase bactericidal responses
   2. Addison's disease
   3. collagen diseases
   4. stimulate ovulation

5. Corticosteroids can be administered by which route(s)? (*Select all that apply.*)
   1. orally
   2. subcutaneously
   3. intravenously
   4. intramuscularly

6. What are three of the most common complications from long-term corticosteroid treatment?
   1. hypoglycemia, weight loss, and cataracts
   2. hypotension, palpitations, and sweating
   3. peptic ulcers, fungal infections, and muscle wasting
   4. anorexia, overstimulated adrenal cortex, and weight gain

7. Mrs. McKensey called the clinic to report that she ran out of her prednisone yesterday. She takes 40 mg a day, and was hoping to get it refilled. What will you tell her?
   1. "There is no reason you can't wait until you see your doctor for your regularly scheduled appointment in a couple of weeks."
   2. "We will call the pharmacy to get your prescription refilled right away; you must be sure to take your dose today."
   3. "You will need to wait until tomorrow for a new prescription. We are really busy today, so call back later."
   4. "The doctor is on vacation until next week, can you call back then?"

PART IV: SEX HORMONES

1. Androgens are used in weak and debilitated patients because they will:
   1. increase sodium retention.
   2. reduce diarrhea, nausea, and vomiting.
   3. restore a positive nitrogen balance.
   4. reverse male pattern baldness.

2. Erythropoiesis is the increase in red blood cell formation that is stimulated with the administration of:
   1. aldosterone.
   2. androgens.
   3. insulin.
   4. estrogens.

3. Estrogens are used for which of the following reasons?
   1. decrease bone growth and decrease serum lipoproteins
   2. reduce urinary retention and prevent prostate cancer
   3. hormone replacement therapy and infertility work-ups
   4. prevent stroke and heart attacks and increase sex drive

4. The hormone given with estrogen in oral contraceptive pills is:
   1. luteinizing hormone.
   2. testosterone.
   3. androgen.
   4. progesterone.

5. How do oral contraceptives work?
   1. prevent ovulation
   2. interfere with egg fertilization
   3. stimulate ovulation
   4. increase uterine bleeding

6. Adverse reactions to oral birth control pills are usually caused by: (*Select all that apply.*)
   1. corticosteroid excess.
   2. corticotropin excess.
   3. progestin excess.
   4. estrogen excess.

7. Why should women over 35 who smoke and who take oral contraceptives be advised to either stop smoking or try other forms of birth control?
   1. They are too old to have children.
   2. They are at increased risk for strokes and blood clots.
   3. They are at increased risk for lung cancer.
   4. They are going to experience decreased effectiveness of the oral contraceptives.

8. Estrogens have the following effect because they are anabolic. (*Select all that apply.*)
   1. decrease in triglycerides
   2. retention of salt
   3. retention of water
   4. increase in cholesterol

9. Generally oral contraceptives are taken for:
   1. 21 days then stop for 7 days.
   2. 28 days then stop for 7 days.
   3. 30 days then stop for 30 days.
   4. 7 days then stop for 21 days.

PART V: THYROID PREPARATIONS

1. Ms. Larkin complains of weight gain, lack of appetite, and a dryness of her skin and hair. She also reports recent difficulty with constipation. The doctor suspects thyroid problems. Thyroid tests would probably show the patient is:
   1. euthyroid.
   2. hyperthyroid.
   3. hypothyroid.
   4. normal thyroid.

2. An increase in thyroid hormone often produces weight loss in patients because:
   1. patients lose their appetites and eat less.
   2. metabolic rate is increased.
   3. patients develop an inability to metabolize food.
   4. metabolic rate is decreased.

3. Thyroid hormones are used in the treatment of which of the following conditions? *(Select all that apply.)*
   1. myxedema
   2. hyperthyroidism
   3. cretinism
   4. nontoxic goiter

4. Drug interactions may occur when patients take thyroid medications and also have which of the following clinical conditions? *(Select all that apply.)*
   1. diabetes mellitus
   2. cardiovascular disease
   3. hypothyroidism
   4. pregnancy

5. Antithyroid preparations are taken when:
   1. the thyroid is enlarged, and the doctor wants to help it return to its normal size.
   2. the synthesis of thyroid hormones must be stimulated.
   3. the patient has very slow reflexes and myxedema.
   4. production of thyroid hormones must be reduced.

6. When patients are taking thyroid medications, they must be instructed to recognize:
   1. hypothyroid and hyperthyroid signs and symptoms.
   2. hypoglycemic and hyperglycemic signs and symptoms.
   3. increased cholesterol and decreased triglyceride effects.
   4. hypothermia and hyperthermia signs and symptoms.

7. Which herbal products are often taken by patients to treat hypothyroidism?
   1. ginkgo and chamomile
   2. bitter melon and garcinia
   3. valerian and passion flower
   4. milk thistle and evening primrose

8. Two antithyroid drugs are:
   1. Tapazole and Levothroid.
   2. Tapazole and propylthiouracil.
   3. propylthiouracil and Eltroxin.
   4. Lugol's iodine and Synthroid.

PART VI: MASTERING HORMONES AND STEROIDS

1. Assume that you have diabetes and have just started to wear an insulin pump. Make a small bag out of a handkerchief and put a rock in it. Tie the bag onto your belt and tuck it into your jeans. Wear it all the time for 2 days. Discuss with your classmates how you felt about this experience. Did you learn anything that might help you in talking to a patient who will wear an insulin pump?

2. Assume that you have just discovered you have diabetes. You do not have any symptoms. You are told by the health care provider that you have to check either your urine or your blood sugar level before every meal. Go to the store and buy 3 different packages of candy, each composed of small pieces. From package #1, take 2 pieces of candy every morning at 9 AM and 1 piece of candy at 5 PM. From package #2, take 3 pieces of candy 1 hour before meals. From package #3, take 1 piece of candy 1 hour before you go to bed. Keep a record of the medications you took and whether you took them on time. If you did not take them on time, explain why. Talk with your classmates and compare experiences. What have you learned about taking medications on a complex dosing schedule? If you were a diabetic, would your blood sugar have been well-managed the way you took the medications or not?

3. What is a sliding-scale insulin dose? This is discussed in your text, but go to the Internet and learn what other things you can about this type of insulin dose. Why would this be a good order for a doctor to write? What problems might develop from using a sliding-scale insulin dose?

4. You are a 34-year-old man and have just been told that you have a low testosterone level (lowT) that will require replacement therapy. Evaluate the different types of testosterone replacement products. What are the pros and cons of each and how would you feel about each of them? What product would you choose to use and why? Find out the cost of each product for one month.

5. You are a busy college girl. You have been using oral birth control pills for several years. When you go to the student health center to renew your prescription, the nurse practitioner notices that you smoke and says that you should stop smoking if you use the pill—or stop taking the pill. You don't want to stop smoking or stop taking the pill. What are your risks if you smoke and take the pill? What are you going to do? Why? Discuss this dilemma with your classmates.

Immunologic Medications

chapter

19

 Go to http://evolve.elsevier.com/edmunds/lpn/ for additional activities and exercises.

PART I: IMMUNOLOGIC AGENTS

1. What is the response of the body when it senses an invasion by a foreign protein?
   1. The body makes antigens.
   2. The body makes toxins.
   3. The body makes antibodies.
   4. The body makes vaccines.

2. What type of immunity occurs when a patient has an illness and then develops antibodies to the causative agent?
   1. passive immunity
   2. naturally acquired active immunity
   3. antigen response
   4. artificially acquired active immunity

3. When a toxin or an antigen is weakened so that it may be given to an individual to provoke antibodies, we say it has been:
   1. artificially acquired.
   2. naturally acquired.
   3. attenuated.
   4. strengthened.

4. When a vaccine is produced in the laboratory and given to individuals to help them develop immunity, the process is called:
   1. artificially acquired active immunity.
   2. artificially acquired passive immunity.
   3. naturally acquired active immunity.
   4. naturally acquired passive immunity.

5. Immunoglobulins are injected into a person who does not have immunity to an antigen such as hepatitis B. This is an example of what type of immunity?
   1. artificially acquired active immunity
   2. naturally acquired active immunity
   3. passive immunity
   4. acquired passive immunity

6. When is it recommended that children get immunized against *Haemophilus influenzae* type B?
   1. birth
   2. 2 months
   3. 12 months
   4. 15 months

7. The most common side effects of immunologic agents are: *(Select all that apply.)*
   1. pain at the injection site.
   2. fever.
   3. localized rash and itching.
   4. a hard lump where the injection was given.

8. Because of the biologic source of some vaccines, occasionally people may be unusually sensitive to immunologic products if they have an allergy to:
   1. eggs or feathers.
   2. grass pollen or trees.
   3. molds.
   4. aspirin or aspartame.

9. Sometimes immunity levels decrease over time. The result of this is that the patient:
   1. remains immune to the organism.
   2. requires a booster immunization to raise immunity level.
   3. eventually develops a mild case of the disease.
   4. will have lifelong immunity as long as there is any antigen-antibody memory in the cells.

10. Which of the following vaccines is recommended to be given at birth?
   1. measles, mumps, rubella
   2. diphtheria, tetanus, pertussis
   3. hepatitis B
   4. inactivated poliovirus

11. Which of these drug(s) is/are used for in vivo testing? *(Select all that apply.)*
    1. coccidioidin
    2. Mantoux
    3. histoplasmin
    4. immune globulin

12. What are the recommended vaccines for children who are starting school?
    1. HepB series, DTap, and varicella
    2. HepB series, MMR, and IPV
    3. HepB series, DTap, MMR, IPV, and varicella
    4. HepB series, IPV, and varicella

PART II: MASTERING IMMUNOLOGIC MEDICATIONS

1. Your hospital has a policy that all health care workers must be immunized against influenza. Your nursing colleague says she doesn't believe in immunizations and is going to refuse to be immunized. Go to the Internet and read about influenza and about why hospitals and many clinics and other agencies require that nurses and physicians be immunized. Explain who is at risk and what the dangers could be to people who are not immunized. What is the risk to their family or others? Do you believe health care agencies should force their employees to get immunized? Talk about this as a group.

2. You know that most states have a law that requires children to have standard immunizations before they can go to school. This is a policy that is monitored every year, and children can't go to school if they are not properly immunized. You have a next-door neighbor whose children are home-schooled. Do they have to be immunized? Who checks to see if they are immunized? Is it a problem if they are not immunized? Talk about this as a group.

3. Your friends at church say that they are not going to let their children be immunized because everyone knows that immunizations cause autism. Go to the Internet and consult the medical literature on this topic. There is much information available. How will you determine which things on the Internet are to be believed? What have you learned that you can share with your classmates? How will you plan to share this information with patients or even your friends at church?

4. How would you learn which immunizations children and adults should take? What is the best source of information about this topic? Looking at the recommendations, do you have all the immunizations you should have? What about your parents or your children?

Topical Medications

e Go to http://evolve.elsevier.com/edmunds/lpn/ for additional activities and exercises.

PART I: TOPICAL PREPARATIONS

1. The patient is suffering from allergic conjunctivitis, and the nurse practitioner orders nedocromil (Alocril). The nurse explains:
   1. "This eye ointment will be effective in relieving your stuffy nose symptoms."
   2. "These eyedrops help to reduce the itchy eye symptoms from allergies by stabilizing the mast cells."
   3. "This eye ointment will relieve your itchy eyes because it has a steroid in it."
   4. "These eyedrops will reduce the pressure in the eye to relieve your symptoms."

2. A new mother is noticing a clear jelly substance in her baby's eyes. The nurse tells her that this is erythromycin (Ilotycin), which the nurse put in the baby's eyes within a few hours after birth. This is done to:
   1. help open the eye to activate the retina.
   2. prevent gonorrheal ophthalmia neonatorum.
   3. improve the baby's visual acuity.
   4. prevent the development of glaucoma.

3. Amanda Moore has been wearing contact lenses for 4 years. She has been studying late at night, and her eyes are very dry. The doctor may decide she needs to use:
   1. a local anesthetic.
   2. antiseptic drops to reduce minor irritation.
   3. artificial tears to lubricate the cornea.
   4. a topical antibiotic to reduce minor infection.

4. Glaucoma medications work in several ways, which include: (*Select all that apply.*)
   1. increasing the outflow of aqueous humor.
   2. increasing intraocular pressure.
   3. blocking the action of acetylcholine.
   4. decreasing the production of aqueous humor.

5. Which of the following herbal products are used for the treatment of mild sunburn? (*Select all that apply.*)
   1. rose hips
   2. aloe
   3. St. John's wort
   4. lavender

6. Topical dermatologic preparations can be used to treat which condition?
   1. pneumonia
   2. glaucoma
   3. lipomas
   4. thyroid nodules

7. Products used for the eye must be labeled:
   1. otic preparation.
   2. otic or topical preparation.
   3. ophthalmic preparation.
   4. ophthalmic or otic preparation.

8. Richard Egan has noted reduced hearing for the last few months. The doctor tells him his ear is filled with wax. The doctor will probably order:
   1. erythromycin (Ilotycin).
   2. carbamide peroxide (Debrox).
   3. hydrogen peroxide.
   4. phenylephrine (Neo-Synephrine).

9. Antiseborrheic shampoo is used to treat which condition?
   1. psoriasis
   2. scabies
   3. herpes simplex
   4. dandruff

10. The nurse is advising the patient on what he needs to use for acne. Which of the following products is used for acne?
    1. acyclovir (Zovirax)
    2. azelaic (Azelex)
    3. benzocaine (Americaine)
    4. alclometasone (Aclovate)

11. The nurse is instructing the patient on how to instill eardrops for the removal of wax using a medication for this purpose. The nurse will explain which of the following?
    1. "Tilt your head at a 45-degree angle and fill the ear canal half-full with the solution and then flush out the solution immediately."
    2. "Tilt your head at a 90-degree angle and fill the ear canal full and leave in for 3 hours before flushing out."
    3. "Tilt your head at a 45-degree angle and fill the ear canal full and leave in for 30 minutes before flushing out."
    4. "Tilt your head at a 90-degree angle and fill the ear canal half-full and leave in for 30 minutes before flushing."

12. When instructing the patient on how to instill eye ointment, the nurse demonstrates the technique and then observes the patient apply the medication:
    1. directly on the eyelid.
    2. to the lower conjunctival sac.
    3. to the upper conjunctival sac.
    4. on a cotton applicator first, then to the inner canthus of the eye.

13. Which of the following topical preparations are used for scabies infections? *(Select all that apply.)*
    1. crotamiton (Eurax)
    2. desonide (Tridesilon)
    3. malathion (Ovide)
    4. permethrin (Elimite)

14. The nurse is caring for a child who is being seen for head lice. The classification of medications used for this problem is usually:
    1. pediculocides.
    2. scabicides.
    3. keratolytics.
    4. emollients.

15. Cauterizing agents are used in the treatment of:
    1. warts.
    2. scabies.
    3. acne.
    4. dandruff.

PART II: MASTERING TOPICAL MEDICATIONS

1. Why is fluorine added to some medications? What does the Internet tell you about this product and why it is often added to some steroids for topical use?

2. What is the major difference between OTC medications you can buy for topical problems and those medications that require a prescription? What is the difference in cost? (You may need to discuss this with your local pharmacist.) Are there herbal products that are used to treat eye, ear, nose, or throat problems?

3. If you had glaucoma, what types of medications would likely be prescribed? How often do patients with glaucoma need to take medication? Does it help? What would happen if they did not take medication?

Vitamins and Minerals

⊖ Go to http://evolve.elsevier.com/edmunds/lpn/ for additional activities and exercises.

PART I: VITAMINS

1. Vitamins are classified according to their solubility. Which vitamins are fat-soluble? (*Select all that apply.*)
   1. vitamin A
   2. vitamin D
   3. vitamin E
   4. vitamin B

2. Although vitamins have been given a letter of the alphabet to identify them, they all have one or more scientific names, depending on the number of chemicals making up that vitamin category. Many prescriptions are written for the scientific name. Match the scientific names of the B vitamins with their commonly used abbreviations.

	Abbreviation		Vitamin
1.	_____	vitamin B_1	a. riboflavin
2.	_____	vitamin B_2	b. pantothenic acid
3.	_____	vitamin B_3	c. thiamine
4.	_____	vitamin B_5	d. folic acid
5.	_____	vitamin B_6	e. niacin
6.	_____	vitamin B_9	f. pyridoxine hydrochloride

3. The nurse is reviewing the foods that are rich in vitamin A for a patient with night blindness. Which foods contain vitamin A? (*Select all that apply.*)
   1. dairy products
   2. eggs
   3. nuts
   4. green vegetables

4. In discussing the use of vitamins with patients, the nurse should include the following in the instructions:
   1. "You should always buy the most expensive vitamins you can find; they are much better for you."
   2. "You can buy any brand of vitamin you wish; the natural and synthetic are usually no different."
   3. "You need to read the label and get the natural vitamins; they are much better than synthetic ones."
   4. "You really should take all the vitamins possible to help you stay well."

5. Vitamin A is important for: (*Select all that apply.*)
   1. helping the eye to adjust to light.
   2. stabilizing the cell membrane.
   3. helping the body resist infection.
   4. producing cholesterol.

6. Why is thiamine important? (*Select all that apply.*)
   1. It is resistant to ultraviolet light.
   2. It is involved in carbohydrate metabolism.
   3. It is water-soluble and functions as a coenzyme.
   4. It is used to treat beriberi.

7. Although vitamins have been given a letter of the alphabet to identify them, they all have one or more scientific names, depending on the number of chemicals making up that vitamin category. Match the scientific name of the vitamin that may appear in the doctor's order or on the prescription with the commonly used abbreviation.

Abbreviation		**Vitamin**
1. _____	vitamin A	a. ascorbic acid
2. _____	vitamin C	b. ergocalciferol
3. _____	vitamin D	c. retinoic acid
4. _____	vitamin E	d. phytonadione

8. *Pellagra* refers to the rare deficiency—occurring most frequently in the U.S., where corn is a major staple food—caused by low levels or lack of which vitamin?
   1. vitamin C
   2. vitamin B (niacin)
   3. vitamin D
   4. vitamin K

9. The symptoms of pellagra include: *(Select all that apply.)*
   1. anorexia.
   2. irritability.
   3. depression.
   4. tinnitus.

10. Good sources of pyridoxine or B_6 include: *(Select all that apply.)*
    1. egg yolk.
    2. muscle meats.
    3. carrots.
    4. wheat.

11. Disorders that can be treated with vitamin D include: *(Select all that apply.)*
    1. convulsions and weight loss.
    2. hypoparathyroidism and hypophosphatemia.
    3. rickets and osteomalacia.
    4. hypervitaminosis and cancer.

12. The preferred route for administration of vitamin K is:
    1. orally and IV.
    2. IV and subcutaneously.
    3. subcutaneously and IM.
    4. orally and IM.

13. Folic acid is used to treat: *(Select all that apply.)*
    1. anemia from alcoholism.
    2. anemia from liver disease.
    3. hyperglycemia from diabetes.
    4. headaches from aneurysms.

14. Many patients now take vitamin D along with other mineral supplements. Symptoms of vitamin D toxicity include:
    1. anorexia, nausea, malaise, and weight loss.
    2. cough, shortness of breath, and rash.
    3. headache, sore throat, and runny nose.
    4. scaly, flaky skin and pruritus.

15. Vitamin C has been used in treating hospitalized patients for years because it can help in a wide variety of conditions, including: *(Select all that apply.)*
    1. treating debilitated or emaciated patients.
    2. strengthening premature infants.
    3. thinning of the blood.
    4. treatment of scurvy.

PART II: MINERALS

1. The major difference between vitamins and minerals is:
   1. vitamins are inorganic and minerals are organic.
   2. minerals are inorganic and vitamins are organic.
   3. minerals are synthetic and vitamins are natural.
   4. vitamins are synthetic and minerals are natural.

2. The Food and Nutrition Board of the National Research Council has established recommended daily intakes for which two minerals?
   1. iodine and manganese
   2. potassium and copper
   3. zinc and magnesium
   4. calcium and iron

3. The three minerals most often missing in the diet in the U.S. are:
   1. calcium, magnesium, and iron.
   2. calcium, zinc, and potassium.
   3. calcium, iron, and iodine.
   4. calcium, iodine, and chloride.

4. Which vitamin should be given with calcium to aid in its absorption?
    1. vitamin A
    2. vitamin D
    3. vitamin K
    4. vitamin E

5. What major mineral in the body is essential for muscular and neurologic activity, repair of skeletal tissues, and activation of enzyme systems?
    1. calcium
    2. zinc
    3. magnesium
    4. iron

6. The nurse notices when taking a blood pressure measurement that the patient has a carpal spasm and reports tingling in that arm. What deficiency may she have?
    1. iron
    2. zinc
    3. calcium
    4. iodine

7. The nurse is giving instructions to a patient taking iron supplements for anemia. The nurse will stress:
    1. "You may develop constipation and/or dark green or black stools with this iron therapy."
    2. "You can take this preparation with food; it may cause sleepiness, so driving may be impaired."
    3. "You can take your antacids with this preparation."
    4. "You could take vitamin E to increase your response to the iron therapy."

8. Which of the following foods are rich in potassium? *(Select all that apply.)*
    1. bananas
    2. tomatoes
    3. apricots
    4. apples

9. Abnormalities of taste and smell, profound lack of interest in food, and rough skin may be associated with overdose of what mineral supplement?
    1. manganese
    2. iron
    3. zinc
    4. copper

PART III: MASTERING VITAMINS AND MINERALS

1. There are many vitamin and mineral supplements on the market. Think about whether you believe everyone should be taking supplements. Go to the Internet and look for the best scientific recommendations about the use of supplements. Which groups or individuals are making the recommendations? Do they agree on their recommendations? How will you decide which groups to believe? Are you surprised by their recommendations?

2. Many young college students report that they never eat fruits and vegetables because they cost too much. What might be the consequences of not eating fruits or vegetables? Which fruits and vegetables cost the least? Talk with your classmates about how you might be successful in encouraging these college students to spend some money to eat fruits and vegetables.

3. Go to a store that sells vitamins or special nutritional supplements. What types of products do they have there? What are the costs for the medications? Are the products directed towards any particular age group? What was your overall impression when you left the store? Discuss your different reactions with your classmates.

Review of Mathematical Principles

e Go to http://evolve.elsevier.com/edmunds/lpn/ for additional activities and exercises.

PART I: REVIEWING MULTIPLICATION FACTS

1. 23
    × 15

2. 213
    × 19

3. 321
    × 11

4. 179
    × 16

5. $200 \times 15 =$

6. $387 \times 35 =$

7. $789 \times 106 =$

8. $2305 \times 3211 =$

9. $21 \times 19 =$

10. $(34)(59) =$

11. $843 \times 79 =$

12. $1798 \times 0 =$

13. $436 \times 212 =$

14. $(79)(64) =$

15. $341 \times 26 =$

16. $2002 \cdot 1007 =$

17. $329,472 \times 3 =$

18. $(246)(835) =$

19. $(404)(103) =$

20. $(601)(47) =$

21. $(333)(58) =$

22. $201 \cdot 34 =$

23. $7530 \cdot 341 =$

24. $47,347 \cdot 6 =$

25. $3400 \times 21 =$

26. $198 \times 4 \times 1 =$

27. $163 \times 3 \times 7 =$

PART II: REVIEWING DIVISION FACTS

Now calculate the following division problems. Do not use the grid unless you must.

1. $3\overline{)213}$

2. $2\overline{)2010}$

3. $3\overline{)70,896}$

4. $4\overline{)2080}$

5. $5\overline{)196,420}$

6. $7\overline{)12,607}$

7. $2880 \div 45 =$

8. $4992 \div 39 =$

9. $8024 \div 136 =$

10. $3\overline{)9034}$

11. $11\overline{)123}$

12. $142 \div 12 =$

13. $25\overline{)25,026}$

14. $17\overline{)3416}$

15. $3429 \div 17 =$

16. $29\overline{)10,859}$

17. $50\overline{)1019}$

18. $428\overline{)10,843}$

19. $100\overline{)1027}$

20. $200,305 \div 2 =$

PART III: WORKING WITH ROMAN NUMERALS

Use the information on the review sheet to change the following Roman numerals into Arabic numerals, and the Arabic numerals to Roman numerals.

1. 11 =

2. 16 =

3. 63 =

4. 77 =

5. 9 =

6. XLIV =

7. XXXII =

8. XV =

9. CDIV =

10. XXVI =

11. 6 =

12. 44 =

13. 49 =

14. 400 =

15. 83 =

16. 40 =

17. XIV =

18. LXII =

19. XCIX =

20. XXX =

21. LXXV =

22. XIV =

PART IV: REVIEW OF BASIC INFORMATION ON FRACTIONS

1. Indicate whether the following are proper fractions (PF), improper fractions (IF), mixed numbers (MN), or complex fractions (CF).

    1. 3/4   5. 8/7

    2. $\dfrac{3\,2/3}{20}$ 6. 2/3

    3. $\dfrac{1/5}{50}$ 7. 8 3/5

    4. 3/1   8. 1/8

2. Change the following improper fractions to mixed numbers.

    1. 13/3   5. 18/7

    2. 25/4   6. 46/15

    3. 3/2   7. 4/3

    4. 6/5   8. 22/3

3. Change the following mixed numbers to improper fractions.

    1. 4 2/3   5. 3 4/5

    2. 6 1/3   6. 1 7/8

    3. 7 3/4   7. 3 1/2

    4. 5 1/12   8. 6 1/2

PART V: PRACTICE ADDING FRACTIONS

Add the following fractions, converting improper fractions to mixed numbers in the lowest terms.

1. $7/8 + 5/8 =$

2. $3/4 + 1/6 =$

3. $1/16 + 5/24 =$

4. $1\,5/6 + 3\,5/9 =$

5. $3/8 + 1/8 =$

6. $3/4 + 2/4 =$

7. $4\,4/5 + 2/5 =$

8. $1\,2/7 + 3\,6/7 =$

9. $6\,3/4 + 2 =$

10. $5/9 + 7/12 =$

11. $1/8 + 3/16 =$

12. $1\,5/9 + 2\,1/3 =$

13. $5\,3/5 + 6\,3/5 =$

14. $6\,7/10 + 4\,1/4 =$

15. $1\,1/2 + 1\,1/4 + 1\,1/8 =$

16. $1\,5/6 + 3\,5/9 =$

17. $5\,1/5 + 2\,2/5 =$

18. $3\,2/7 + 4/7 =$

19. $1\,3/4 + 3\,3/8 =$

20. $4\,5/6 + 2\,1/8 =$

PART VI: PRACTICE SUBTRACTING FRACTIONS

1. $5/8 - 3/8 =$

2. $5/6 - 7/9 =$

3. $4\,1/4 - 3\,3/8 =$

4. $7/10 - 3/10 =$

5. $5/18 - 3/18 =$

6. $5/6 - 1/4 =$

7. $7/8 - 7/40 =$

8. $3/4 - 1/2 =$

9. $1/4 - 1/5 =$

10. $3 - 1/4 =$

11. $7 - 3/5 =$

12. $5 - 1\,2/3 =$

13. $4 - 3\,1/8 =$

14. $3\,1/3 - 1\,2/3 =$

15. $6\,3/10 - 3\,7/10 =$

PART VII: PRACTICE MULTIPLYING FRACTIONS

Make equivalent fractions.

1. $1/6 = $ _____ $/12$

2. $2/3 = $ _____ $/15$

3. $7/9 = 56/$ _____

4. $1/7 = $ _____ $/28$

5. $3/9 = $ _____ $/27$

Multiply the following fractions, converting to the lowest terms, and changing improper fractions to mixed numbers.

6. $2/5 \bullet 7/8 =$

7. $1/2 \bullet 4/3 \bullet 1/2 =$

8. $2/3 \bullet 9/4 =$

9. $2/7 \bullet 49/4 =$

10. $11/12 \bullet 12/11 =$

11. $3 \bullet 1/9 =$

12. $(11/17) (34/11) (1/2) =$

13. $(2/5) (25/10) (3/8) =$

14. $(1/27) (54/2) (18/1) =$

15. $(9) (1/3) (3/4) (1/5) =$

PART VIII: PRACTICE DIVIDING FRACTIONS

Divide the following fractions, reducing to lowest terms.

1. $4/5 \div 3/10 =$

2. $8 \div 2/3 =$

3. $5/9 \div 3/4 =$

4. $6/7 \div 3 =$

5. $3/8 \div 6/7 =$

6. $1/6 \div 1/3 =$

7. $4/6 \div 2/3 =$

8. $5/9 \div 2/5 =$

9. $3\,1/2 \div 2\,2/3 =$

10. $4\,2/3 \div 1/3 =$

11. $1\,2/3 \div 2\,1/2 =$

12. $6\,1/2 \div 2 =$

13. $1\,3/4 \div 5\,1/4 =$

14. $3/5 \div 3/10 =$

15. $2/5 \div 5/8 =$

PART IX: PRACTICE WITH DECIMAL FRACTIONS

Change the following decimals to fractions:

1. 0.807 =

2. 0.0207 =

3. 0.12347 =

4. 0.666 =

5. 0.01 =

6. 1.3 =

Convert to common fractions or mixed numbers in lowest terms:

7. 0.202 =

8. 3.14 =

9. 103.004 =

10. 0.75 =

11. 0.40 =

12. 2.125 =

13. 0.6 =

14. 0.33 =

15. 0.26 =

Find:

16. 7.456 + .923 + 1.04 + 7.3 =

17. 31.8579 + 11.264 + 32.79 =

18. 17.77 − 6.5 =

19. 4.03 − 2.1856 =

20. 2.231 × 0.32 =

21. 213 × 1.28 =

22. 0.172 × 0.012 × 12 =

23. 0.00572 × 100 =

24. 100 × 0.0453 =

25. 9.128 ÷ 0.028 =

26. 36 ÷ 0.09 =

PART X: PRACTICE WITH RATIOS AND PERCENTS

Change to percents.

1.   .32 =

2.   2 1/6 =

3.   2/5 =

Change to decimal fractions.

4.   67% =

5.   105% =

6.   1/4% =

7.   Change 14 2/7% to a common fraction in its lowest terms:

8.   Express 233 1/3% as a mixed number:

9.   Write 4 1/5 as a decimal:

10. Write 48% as a decimal:

11. Write 15% as a fraction reduced to its lowest terms:

12. Write 1.79 as a percent:

13. Write 1.25 as a percent:

14. Write 2 1/4 as a percent:

Ratios:

15. Write a ratio that expresses 10,000 people to a mile:

16. Ratio of 1 stamp for every dollar of purchase:

17. 7 to 4:

18. 2 eggs to 1 person:

19. 1/2 to 1/5:

20. 24 cans to 2 cases:

21. 2 feet to 7 feet:

22. 12 to 1:

23. 1 1/2 to 1 3/4:

24. 1000 square miles per person:

25. 3000 raindrops per 10 yards:

PART XI: PRACTICE WITH PROPORTIONS

Calculate the following, rounding decimals to the nearest hundredth:

1. $\dfrac{3.6}{2.9} = \dfrac{x}{4.3}$

2. $\dfrac{6.15}{12} = \dfrac{17.39}{x}$

3. $\dfrac{19.056}{x} = \dfrac{3.72}{16.57}$

4. $\dfrac{5}{6} = \dfrac{x}{42}$

5. $\dfrac{3}{4} = \dfrac{9}{x}$

6. $\dfrac{x}{8} = \dfrac{12}{48}$

7. $\dfrac{7}{x} = \dfrac{8}{120}$

8. $\dfrac{1\frac{1}{2}}{\frac{1}{2}} = \dfrac{x}{4}$

9. $\dfrac{\frac{2}{3}}{\frac{10}{15}} = \dfrac{4}{x}$

10. $\dfrac{x}{1\frac{1}{5}} = \dfrac{\frac{35}{42}}{\frac{4}{3}}$

11. $\dfrac{\frac{5}{9}}{x} = \dfrac{\frac{3}{4}}{1\frac{28}{35}}$

12. $0.2 : 1 :: 0.6 : x$

13. $\dfrac{\frac{1}{48}}{\frac{1}{32}} = \dfrac{x}{2}$

14. $\dfrac{0.0002}{1} = \dfrac{x}{2}$

15. $10 : 2 :: 80 : x$

Mathematical Equivalents Used in Pharmacology

Go to http://evolve.elsevier.com/edmunds/lpn/ for additional activities and exercises.

PART I: COMMON HOUSEHOLD AND APOTHECARY SYSTEMS

1. Change 5 quarts to pints.

2 Change 6 gallons to quarts.

Give abbreviations for the following units.

3. cubic centimeter _____

4. ounce _____

5. grain _____

6. kilogram _____

7. gram _____

8. pint _____

9. milligram _____

10. microgram _____

11. milliliter _____

PART II: METRIC SYSTEM

Calculate the answers to these problems using the metric system.

1. Change 3.4 meters to centimeters.

2. Change 5 meters to centimeters.

3. Change 4 meters to millimeters.

4. 5 g = _____ mg

5. 2000 cc = _____ L

6. 1000 mL = _____ L

7. 1 mL = _____ cc

8. 100 mg = _____ g

9. 1 mg = _____ mcg

10. 5 g = _____ mg

11. 1200 mg = _____ g

12. 1.5 L = _____ mL

13. _____ L = 3000 mL

14. _____ L = 250 mL

15. 0.04 g = _____ mg

16. _____ g = 1.4 kg

17. 150 mg = _____ g

18. 1 kg = _____ g

19. 1 mcg = _____ mg

20. _____ cm = 0.02 m

21. _____ m = 1000 cm

22. 10 L = _____ decaliter

PART III: CONVERTING BETWEEN APOTHECARY AND METRIC SYSTEMS

Calculate the answers to these problems.

1. 0.1 mg = _____ g

2. 15 mg = gr _____

3. 60 mg = _____ g

4. 1 g = gr _____

5. _____ mg = gr 1/150

6. 0.016 g = gr _____

7. 60 mg = gr _____

8. gr 1/2 = _____ g

9. gr 1/100 = _____ mg

10. gr viiss = _____ g

11. gr 1/6 = _____ mg

12. 0.1 g = _____ mg

13. 0.01 g = _____ gr

14. 0.5 g = _____ gr = _____ mg

15. 2.5 kg = _____ lb = _____ g

16. 100 mg = gr _____

17. gr 1/16 = _____ g

18. gr 1/4 = _____ g = _____ mg

19. gr 1/15 = _____ mg

20. 0.008 g = gr _____

PART IV: USING CELSIUS AND FAHRENHEIT SCALES

Calculate the following answers, rounding to the nearest tenth degree.

1. 40° C = _____ ° F

2. 99° F = _____ ° C

3. 36.6° C = _____ ° F

4. 45° C = _____ ° F

5. 104° F = _____ ° C

6. 37.5° C = _____ ° F

7. 101° F = _____ ° C

8. 30° C = _____ ° F

9. 95° F = _____ ° C

10. 113° F = _____ ° C

Calculating Drug Dosages

 Go to http://evolve.elsevier.com/edmunds/lpn/ for additional activities and exercises.

PART I: PRACTICE COMPUTING ORAL DOSAGES

Calculate the following involving tablets, capsules, or liquids.

1. Desired: Aspirin 500 mg orally every 4 hours
    Available: Aspirin 0.5 g/tablet
    How many tablets per dose? _____

2. Desired: Elixir phenobarbital 60 mg orally every 4 hours
    Available: Phenobarbital 15 mg/5 mL
    How many mL per dose? _____

3. Desired: Chloral hydrate syrup 500 mg orally three times daily
    Available: Chloral hydrate syrup 500 mg/5 mL
    How many mL per dose? _____

4. Desired: Metronidazole 750 mg orally stat and 500 mg orally every 8 hours x 7 days
    Available: Metronidazole 250 mg capsules
    How many capsules per stat dose?_____
    How many doses total for stat dose + 7 days' worth?_____

5. Desired: Elixir ferrous sulfate 600 mg orally three times daily with meals
    Available: Elixir ferrous sulfate 300 mg/10 mL
    How many mL per dose? _____

6. Desired: KCl 40 mEq orally four times daily
    Available: KCl 20 mEq/15 mL
    How many mL per dose? _____

7. Desired: Doxycycline 0.3 g orally every 12 hours x 8 days
    Available: Doxycycline 150 mg capsules
    Number of capsules per dose? _____
    Total number of capsules to be given? _____

8. Desired: Amoxicillin 500 mg orally every 6 hours x 4 days
    Available: Amoxicillin 250 mg per tablet
    How many tablets per dose? _____

9. Desired: Guaifenesin 300 mg orally daily
    Available: Guaifenesin 100 mg/5 mL
    How many mL per dose? _____

10. Desired: Theophylline elixir 100 mg orally twice daily
    Available: Theophylline elixir 0.05 g/5 mL
    How many mL/dose? _____
    How many g/dose? _____

Practice Reading Labels

11. Order is for diltiazem HCl 60 mg orally twice daily.

    1.   What is available? Look at the label to find this.

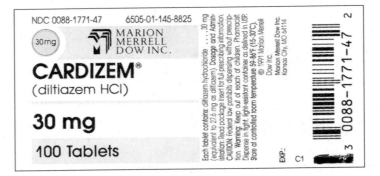

    2.   How many tablets should be given per dose?

    3.   How many tablets will be given in a 24-hour period?

    4.   What is the total amount (mg) of medication given in 24 hours?

12. Order is for Ceclor 0.5 g orally three times daily.

    1.   What is available? Look at the label to find this.

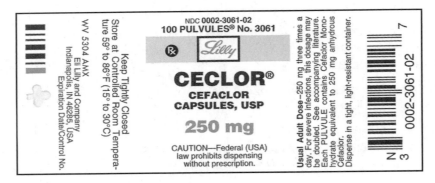

    2.   How many tablets should be given per dose?

    3.   How many tablets will be given in a 24-hour period?

    4.   What is the total amount (mg) of medication given in 24 hours?

13. Order is for Principen 750 mg orally every 8 hours.

    1. What is available? Look at the label to find this.

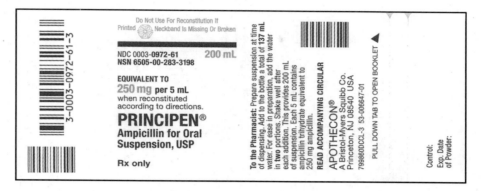

    2. How many mL should be given per dose?

    3. How many mL will be given in a 24-hour period?

    4. What is the total amount (mg) of medication given in 24 hours?

14. Order is for digoxin 0.25 mg IV daily.

    1. What is available? Look at the label to find this.

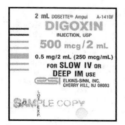

    2. How many mL should be given per dose?

    3. How many mL will be given in a 24-hour period?

    4. What is the total amount (mg) of medication given in 24 hours?

15. Order is for heparin 5000 units subcutaneously twice daily.

    1. What is available? Look at the label to find this.

       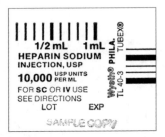

    2. How many mL should be given per dose?

    3. How many mL will be given in a 24-hour period?

    4. What is the total amount (units) of medication given in 24 hours?

16. Order is for hydrochlorothiazide (HydroDIURIL) 25 mg orally every 6 hours.

    1. What is available? Look at the label to find this.

       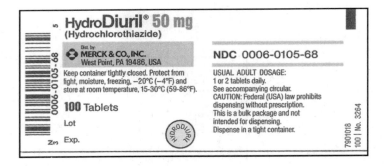

    2. How many tablets should be given per dose?

    3. How many tablets will be given in a 24-hour period?

    4. What is the total amount (mg) of medication given in 24 hours?

PART II: PRACTICE COMPUTING PARENTERAL DOSAGES

Calculate the following problems for parenteral dosages.

1. Desired: Morphine sulfate 10 mg IV
   Available: Morphine sulfate 16 mg/mL
   How many mL per dose? _____

2. Desired: Penicillin G 400,000 units IM
   Available: Penicillin G 1,000,000 units/5 mL
   How many mL per dose? _____

3. Desired: Atropine sulfate 0.1 mg IV
   Available: Atropine sulfate 0.05 mg/mL
   How many mL per dose? _____

4. Desired: Demerol 50 mg IM stat
   Available: Demerol 100 mg/2 mL
   How many mL per dose? _____

5. Desired: Tigan 200 mg IM every 8 hours prn nausea
   Available: Tigan 0.1 g/mL
   How many mL per dose? _____

6. Desired: Aminophylline 0.25 g IM every 4 hours prn wheezing
   Available: Aminophylline 500 mg/2 mL
   How many mL per dose? _____

7. Desired: Procaine penicillin G 500,000 units IM twice daily
   Available: Procaine penicillin G 300,000 units/mL
   How many mL per dose? _____

8. Desired: Dilaudid 4 mg orally every 4 hours prn pain
   Available: Dilaudid 2 mg/mL
   How many mL per dose? _____

Practice Reading Labels

9. Order is for heparin 6000 units subcutaneously three times daily.

   1. What is available? Look at the label to find this.

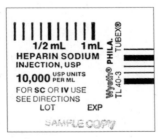

   2. How many mL should be given per dose?

   3. How many mL will be given in a 24-hour period?

   4. What is the total amount (units) of medication given in 24 hours?

10. Order is for Kanamycin 15 mg/kg/day in three divided doses (every 8 hours) IV. Patient weighs 50 kg. Calculate mg desired: 15 mg/kg × 50 kg = 750 mg desired.

    1. What is available? Look at the label to find this.

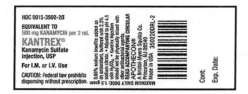

    2. How many mL will be given in a 24-hour period?

    3. Divide into three equal doses. How many mg are given per dose?

11. Order is for meperidine (Demerol) 30 mg IM stat.

    1. What is available? Look at the label to find this.

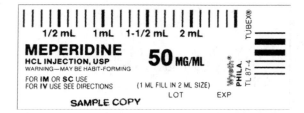

    2. How many mL will be given per dose?

PART III: PRACTICE COMPUTING INSULIN DOSAGES

State the insulin you would use and calculate the following problems for insulin:

1. Order: 45 units NPH (isophane insulin suspension) U-100 1 hour before breakfast daily.

Syringe	Type Insulin and Name	Amount
U-100	_____	_____

2. Order: 38 units Lente insulin U-100 (insulin zinc suspension) 1 hour before breakfast daily.

Syringe	Type Insulin and Name	Amount
U-100	_____	_____

3. Order: 30 units PZI (protamine zinc insulin) U-100 and 20 units regular (Iletin) insulin U-100 30 minutes at breakfast daily.

Syringe	Type Insulin and Name	Amount
U-100	U-100 PZI and regular	_____

4. Order: 40 units regular (Iletin) insulin U-100 30 minutes before meals three times daily.

Syringe	Type Insulin and Name	Amount
U-100	_____	_____

5. Order: 25 units regular (crystalline zinc) insulin U-100 and NPH (isophane insulin suspension) U-100 40 units 30 minutes before breakfast daily.

Syringe	Type Insulin and Name	Amount
U-100	U-100 NPH and regular	_____

Practice Reading Labels

6. Read the insulin label and answer the following questions:

   Mrs. Bennie has had an allergic reaction to NPH Iletin pork insulin. The health care provider has changed the insulin to NPH Humulin insulin 55 units subcutaneously daily before breakfast.

   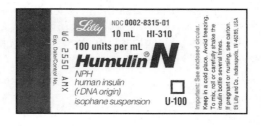

   1. What is the source of insulin?

   2. Is this the correct source of insulin?

   3. How many units per mL?

   4. Using a U-100 insulin syringe, how many units would you give?

7. Order reads regular insulin 10 units and NPH insulin 25 units subcutaneously every day at 8 AM for Mrs. Bennie.

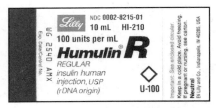
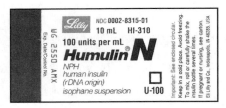
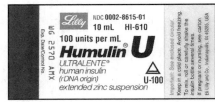
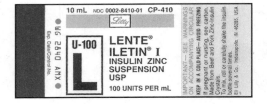
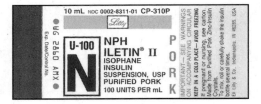

1. Study the labels above. Which of these bottles would the nurse use to draw up regular insulin?

2. Which of these bottles would the nurse use to draw up NPH insulin?

3. What is the total amount of insulin in the syringe?

4. List in order the steps the nurse would take to draw up the insulin.
   1. Wipe skin with alcohol.
   2. Draw up regular insulin.
   3. Inject insulin after selecting site.
   4. Draw up NPH insulin.
   5. Document the medication.

   _____, _____, _____, _____, _____

PART IV: PRACTICE COMPUTING IV INFUSION RATES AND TIMES

1. The physician orders 1000 mL 5% dextrose in water (D_5W) to be administered in 4 hours. Drop factor is 10 gtt/mL. Calculate the following.
    1. The number of minutes the medication is to flow

    2. The number of milliliters the patient will receive per minute

    3. The number of drops the patient will receive per minute

2. Give 1000 mL D_5W at 30 gtt/min. Drop factor is 15 gtt/mL. Calculate the following.
    1. The total number of drops to be given

    2. The total number of minutes to flow

    3. The total time for infusion in hours and minutes

3. Give 400 mL lactated Ringer's solution in 3 hours. The drop factor is 15 gtt/mL. Calculate the following.
    1. The total number of minutes to flow

    2. The number of mL the patient will receive per minute

    3. The number of drops per minute

4. Infuse 500 mL blood in 2 hours. Administration set has a drop factor of 10. How many drops per minute?

5. The patient was given 1000 mL normal saline in 5 hours. What was the rate of administration (flow rate) if the drop factor was 15?

6. Determine the flow rate for IV administration of 1200 mL to be given at rate of 3 mL/min. Drop factor is 15.

7. Give an infant 60 mL of IV D_5W at 0.5 mL/min. Drop factor is 60. Calculate the following.
    1. Determine the total number microdrops.

    2. Determine the total number minutes of flow.

    3. Determine the hours and minutes the solution is to flow.

    4. Determine the flow rate.

8. Give an infant 90 mL IV infusion at rate of 30 microgtt/min. Drop factor is 60. Calculate the following.
    1. The total number of microdrops to be given

    2. The total number of minutes infusion is to flow

    3. The total number of hours and minutes the solution is to flow

PART V: PRACTICE CALCULATING PEDIATRIC DOSAGES

Using Clark's rule, calculate the following dosages for the pediatric orders, assuming normal adult weight of 150 lbs or 68 kg:

1. Morphine 1 mg for a 25-lb 18-month-old

2. Aminophylline 0.5 g for a 17-kg 6-year-old

3. Gentamicin 80 mg for a 28-lb 22-month-old

4. Cleocin 200 mg for a 24-kg 9-year-old

5. Kantrex 0.5 g for a 22-lb 10-month-old

6. Phenobarbital sodium 4 mg for a 12-kg 12-month-old

Use the BSA nomogram on p. 45 of the study guide to determine the child's BSA in square meters.

7. Adult dose: Acetaminophen 500 mg
    Child's height: 30 inches
    Child's weight: 20 lbs
    Child's age: 12 mos

8. Adult dose: Phenobarbital 50 mg
    Child's height: 34 inches
    Child's weight: 26 lbs
    Child's age: 24 mos

9. Adult dose: Warfarin 2 mg
    Child's height: 35 inches
    Child's weight: 32 lbs
    Child's age: 3 yrs

10. Adult dose: Prednisone 20 mg
    Child's height: 52 inches
    Child's weight: 60 lbs
    Child's age: 8 yrs

11. Adult dose: Furosemide 40 mg
    Child's height: 26 inches
    Child's weight: 15 lbs
    Child's age: 6 mos

Practice Reading Labels

12. Order: Cefadroxil (Duricef) 500 mg orally every 12 hours
    Child's weight: 20 lbs
    Child's recommended drug dosage: 30 mg/kg/day

    1. What is available? Look at the label to find this out.

    2. How many lbs per kg? Convert 20 lbs into kg.

    3. What is the dosage range for this child?

    4. Is the prescribed drug dose within safe parameters?

    5. How many mL per dose?

    6. How many mL in a 24-hour period?

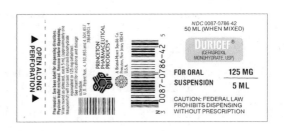

PART VI: MASTERING DRUG CALCULATIONS

1. The physician has ordered 0.5 g of ampicillin IM. The label reads "1 g ampicillin powder. For IM use, must be reconstituted with 3.5 mL of diluent. Resulting diluent contains 250 mg ampicillin per 1 mL." How much of the diluted medication do you administer to the patient?

2. The order is for digoxin (Lanoxin) 0.375 mg IV. The medication comes in 0.5 mg in 2 mL. How much of the medication should be administered?

3. Mrs. Bodkins, age 70, has type 2 diabetes and has been admitted with dehydration, confusion, vomiting, and hypotension. She has not taken her insulin and has not been eating. Her blood glucose level is 530 mg/dL. The order is to start an IV with 1000 mL of 0.45 normal saline, then give 7 units of regular insulin IV push stat, and follow it with an insulin drip of 7 units per hour. The medication available is Humulin Regular 100 units per mL. If you prepared an insulin drip of 50 units of regular insulin in 50 mL of NS, how much would you infuse in 1 hour?

4. A vial of penicillin G aqueous contains 5,000,000 units (U) per vial. It may be reconstituted with different amounts of diluent to produce different concentrations according to the following.

Diluent	Concentration/mL
23 mL	200,000 U
18 mL	250,000 U
8 mL	500,000 U
3 mL	1,000,000 U

If you dilute the 5,000,000 U vial with 23 mL, how many units of penicillin are in each milliliter?

5. The pediatrician orders that an infant is to be given 350 mg Ceftin IM every 6 hours. The medication comes in 220 mg/mL. How much should the nurse give?